Journal of Elder Policy

Also from Westphalia Press
westphaliapress.org

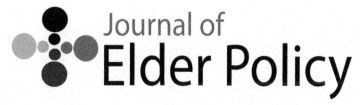

Journal of
Elder Policy

VOLUME 1, NUMBER 2 • SPRING 2021

Eva Kahana PhD, *Editor-In-Chief*

Westphalia Press
An imprint of Policy Studies Organization

Journal of Elder Policy
Vol. 1, No. 2 • Spring 2021

Westphalia Press
An imprint of Policy Studies Organization
1527 New Hampshire Ave., NW
Washington, D.C. 20036
info@ipsonet.org

ISBN: 978-1-63723-903-2

Cover and interior design by Jeffrey Barnes
jbarnesbook.design

Daniel Gutierrez-Sandoval, Executive Director
PSO and Westphalia Press

Updated material and comments on this edition
can be found at the Westphalia Press website:
www.westphaliapress.org

CONTENTS

Terry Hokenstad, PhD, Case Western Reserve University
Distinguished University Professor Emeritus, Ralph S. and Dorothy P. Schmitt Professor Emeritus, Jack, Joseph and Morton Mandel School of Applied Social Sciences, Professor of Global Health, School of Medicine
Research Interests: comparative service delivery systems (focused on the developed world); policies and programs promoting active ageing; age friendly cities

Robert (Bob) Hudson, PhD, Boston University
Professor of Social Welfare Policy
Research Interests: Politics and policies of aging; cross-national welfare state development; design and implementation of social policies

Nancy Kropf, PhD, Georgia State University
Dean, Perimeter College, Professor of Social Work
Research Interests: late life caregiving relationships, geriatric workforce issues, evidence based practice and interventions

Nina Kohn, JD, Syracuse University
Associate Dean of Online Education, David M. Levy L'48 Professor of Law
Research Interests: elder law and the civil rights of older adults and persons with diminished cognitive capacity, financial exploitations of the elderly, elder abuse legislation, ageism

Carol Musil, PhD, RN, FAAN, FGSA, Case Western Reserve University
The Marvin E. and Ruth Durr Denekas Professor of Nursing
Research Interests: caregiving; families; intergenerational relationships: mental health; depressive symptoms, grandparenthood

Holger Pfaff, PhD, University of Cologne
Professor, Institute for Medical Sociology, Health Services Research, and Rehabilitation Science (IMVR), Faculty of Human Sciences, Faculty of Medicine
Research Interests: health literacy, work and aging, health care systems

Jill Quadagno, PhD, Florida State University
Mildren and Claude Pepper Eminent Scholar Emerita, Research Associate, Pepper Institute on Aging and Public Policy
Research Interests: health policy, long term care, race/ethnic inequality

Karen A. Roberto, PhD, Virginia Tech
University Distinguished Professor, Center for Gerontology, Director, Institute for Society, Culture, & Environment
Research Interests: family relationships and dementia caregiving, elder abuse, rural health and aging

Richard Settersten, PhD, Oregon State University
Barbara E. Knudson Professor of Human Development and Family Sciences and Head of the School of Social and Behavioral Health Sciences
Research Interests: life transitions; social relationships; age; parenthood; social policy; inequality

Robyn Stone, DrPH, LeadingAge
Senior Vice President of Research and Co-Director, LeadingAge LTSS Center @UMass Boston
Research Interests: long term services and supports policy and delivery, affordable senior housing, aging services workforce, health and LTSS integration

Joseph White, PhD, Case Western Reserve University
Luxenberg Family Professor of Public Policy, Professor of Political Science and Professor of Population and Quantitative Health Sciences; Director, Center for Policy Studies
Research Interests: Comparing health care systems in the U.S. and other rich democracies; Social Security and Medicare; Policies to control health care spending

CASE WESTERN RESERVE UNIVERSITY ADVISORY COMMITTEE

Grover C. Gilmore, PhD
Dean Mandel School of Applied Social Sciences, Professor of Psychology

Brian Gran, PhD
Professor of Sociology and Law

David Hammack, PhD
Hiram C. Haydn Professor of History Emeritus

Sharona Hoffman, JD
Edgar A. Hahn Professor of Law; Professor of Bioethics
sharonahoffman.com

Diana Morris, PhD
Florence Cellar Associate Professor of Gerontological Nursing, Director Center on Aging and Health

J. B. Silvers, PhD
John R. Mannix Medical Mutual of Ohio Professor of Health Care Finance, Professor, Banking and Finance

Kurt Stange, MD, PhD
Distinguished University Professor, Gertrude Donnelly Hess, Professor of Oncology Research, Professor of Family Medicine & Community Health, Epidemiology & Biostatistics and Sociology

Improving the End-of-Life Experience of Elderly Patients and Their Families: Policy and Practice Fall Short of Providing Comfort and Support

Eva Kahana, PhD, Editor-in-Chief

This editorial is dedicated to my late husband Boaz Kahana, and to older patients facing the end of life in acute care hospitals.

On November 6, 2020, I lost my husband, soulmate, and research collaborator of 58 years, Dr. Boaz Kahana. Boaz was an eminent scholar, a prize-winning and devoted teacher and mentor, and a prince of a man. He retired from his position as Professor of Psychology at Cleveland State University in December of 2019, less than a year before his death. During his brief retirement, he was completing a book for first-generation college students, studying foreign languages, and reading science magazines. He died at one of the premier hospitals in the US. He was 86 years old and a long term, 21-year survivor of Whipple surgery. He fought a valiant battle to survive. Our primary care doctor called me to offer condolences and told me that my "fierce advocacy" and involvement in Boaz's care is likely to have extended his life.

As I introduce the second volume of the *Journal of Elder Policy* in the midst of grieving for Boaz and the persistent global trauma of COVID 19, I would like to draw on my life experiences to explore the liminal areas between old age, ill health, deficiencies in health care practices, and social supports as people approach the end of life. I will also briefly touch on challenges of bereaved elders. My major concern relates to the questions: How are policies, like those presented and discussed in the *Journal of Elder Policy* and others, translated into practices, and how do elderly individuals and their families experience prevailing practices?

The articles in this volume span a broad spectrum of late life challenges and policy solutions that might address these challenges. I am hoping in this editorial to relate them to the lived experience of nearing the end of life. I focus on our common vulnerability and common humanity, which transcend specific policy issues. Robert Binstock (1989) explained the complex interfaces between public policy and implementation. He noted that the hierarchical chains through which policies are carried out are extensive. In relation to health and social service programs, he suggested that it is the employee of the service organization who implements policies that are designed by policymakers and experienced by clients.

As the powerful waves of grief wash over me, suddenly the abstractions of intellectual inquiry about social policies fade into the background. It is only intimate memories and the desire to improve the dying and the bereavement ex-

1   doi: 10.18278/jep.1.2.1

periences of other human beings that lift me up. I feel that it is useful to put the abstract and scholarly articles we publish in a human context of lived experience to fully appreciate their relevance and contributions. My comments in this editorial encompass both observations of my husband's final days and my own experiences with being an elder coping with loss and the altered social status of widowhood.

Shortly after Boaz's death and just before Thanksgiving, I experienced a shock when I received a well-meaning call from a volunteer, who was affiliated with a local community organization. She told me that as a recent widow, I was entitled to a free meal that could be delivered to me for Thanksgiving. While it is nice that this service exists, especially for older adults who may face food security issues during this pandemic, there was little empathy for my grief in this interaction. The focus was only on implementation of service delivery reflecting a social policy.

I thanked the caller and told her that I would not be needing this benefit and hung up the phone with tears trickling down my face. In my mind flashed vivid images of Thanksgivings past when Boaz and I invited to our home our domestic and international students who could not travel home for the Holiday. I remembered welcoming them in a spirit of gratitude as important guests in our home partaking in a homemade meal at a festive table. Not only did I lose my best friend and partner for almost 60 years, but my interaction with this service provider made me feel like I was reduced to a lonely charity case looking for a free Thanksgiving dinner.

As scholars, we advocate for better social policies for elders, but seldom think of what it feels like to be on the receiving end of entitlements. Do our policies take into account the rich life histories of older care recipients? Are emotional and spiritual needs considered by policy makers and service providers? How much respect do service recipients receive?

In his book *Being Mortal* (2014), Atul Gawande offers important insights about the disconnect between older adults' needs and aspirations near the end of their lives, and health care providers' understandings of those needs. During patients' final stays at a hospital or nursing home, where most elders die, there is little communication about the fears, options, and desires of patients. Our policies have evolved to soliciting advance directives from patients, but we do little to ensure that they fully understand the implications of such directives.

In my husband's case, a well-meaning palliative care doctor stopped by his room soon after his arrival to the hospital. The doctor made conversation about the science magazines that my husband was reading. As almost an afterthought, he asked my husband if, "in the unlikely event of his health further declining, would he still want interventions to extend his life?" The eternal optimist, Boaz replied, "Of course, I would want to get all the help I could get." The doctor did not explain the nature of end-of-life interventions he had in mind, nor the likelihood of their success. When the time came to make final decisions, my sons and I opted against heroic measures to extend Boaz's life. Many doctors do not explain that heroic measures may extend life, but they do not always provide quality of life for the time that the person is kept alive.

Boaz was hospitalized on the recommendation of our competent and caring primary care doctor to try to figure out what was causing the extreme fatigue and weakness that he had been experiencing for months. He died in the hospital 10 days later. It was good that during Boaz's final hours, our sons and I were allowed to be with him. Up until that point, only I had been able to visit. During the pandemic, meaningful contact of hospitalized patients and family members has been curtailed. The hospital where Boaz was a patient only allowed one designated family member to visit due to understandable concerns about the spread of COVID-19.

My personal experience with an end-of-life crisis for my husband, and the way the hospital service system works is not unique to me. Many families over this past year have experienced close up the workings of the health care system during COVID-19. They too have confronted end of life decision-making within a system that aims at harmonizing services, but often misses the mark as bureaucratic structures and service policies prevent them from achieving the goals of compassionate care (Youngson, 2011; Kneafsey et al., 2016).

As we advocate for better social policies to protect elders, experts typically rely on logic and results of prior studies. The quality of medical care is seldom viewed through the patient's eyes (Gerteis, 1993). Additionally, while qualitative studies exist for patient experiences, it does not seem that these studies are used as evidence for the development of policy—whether it is because they are based on "subjective" experiences or small study samples. In a sense, they are not viewed as rigorous research, despite providing a window into what it is like to be on the receiving end of healthcare practices and health policies. In the current climate of health care delivery, financial considerations and funding protocols play important roles. These evolving algorithms provide little incentive or even room for patient centered care (Constrand et al., 2014).

Medical care has increasingly less to do with caring for patients and more to do with efficient delivery of services with the patient, considered as the object of care delivery, rather than as a suffering human being (Salamon, 2008; Sweet, 2013). A person lying in an uncomfortable bed, hooked up to IV, unable to eat and too weak to use a regular bathroom, is reduced to being a passive recipient of care. Seriously ill patients are not in a position to ask questions and articulate their fears of abandonment when there are no family members present. Helping to maintain the human dignity and comfort of the patient, such as brushing teeth and having a well-groomed appearance, does not seem to be high on care providers busy do list (Henderson et al., 2009). In addition to being hungry and weak, Boaz also felt cold, particularly at night. I brought him sweaters, gloves and a hat, so he would be more comfortable. It was my task, before leaving in the evening, to help him put on the warm clothing. I wondered about the precarious the position of other lonely older patients hospitalized without access to family. Doctors and nurses are seldom willing or able to discuss patient fears, concerns, and comfort.

Boaz had undergone a successful procedure to place a pancreatic stent during the third day after his hospitalization and we felt optimistic about his recovery. This impression was reinforced by the physician's demeanor. However, he encountered complications as they tried for five days to establish an artificial nutrition regimen. He was not provided any food by mouth during this period. He was clearly distressed, uncomfortable, and increasingly agitated. He whispered to me fearfully: How long will they starve me? I had no answers for him. I could only offer to check with his nurses and doctors. Indeed, doctors visited Boaz in teams of 4 or 5 specialists at a time. They largely conferred among themselves and different nutrition teams (IV vs. tube feeding), and appeared to each prefer their specific strategies. The doctors visiting gave little indication of Boaz's prospects. They did not address him directly and no one inquired about the discomfort he was experiencing.

Boaz retained his mental acuity until his final moments. As he became too weak to talk I gave him paper and pen, so he could write down what he wanted. He would ask that I set his watch to the right time including the day. He wanted the dignity of being oriented to time. He wrote "Thursday," the day before he died. He was reminding me what day of the week to set his watch to. This makes me think of the importance of protecting and ensuring dignity, close to the end of life.

There was no indication Thursday evening that Boaz's condition worsened. I arrived Friday morning shocked to find various staff surrounding him. I was told to wait outside as they tried to suction out a pill that Boaz aspirated. My impression was that they had succeeded and I was not informed that his condition turned critical. A representative of Hospice came by later Friday morning and asked if I would like to take Boaz home so he could receive comfort care and spend time surrounded by family. Again, there was no mention of his imminent demise and I did not ask how long he had. I enthusiastically embraced the idea of bringing him home. Since he was now viewed as a hospice patient, our sons were allowed to visit. They both arrived expeditiously.

In the early afternoon, a physical therapist came by and did some maneuvers of Boaz's body. During this process Boaz's breathing became labored. Nurses rushed in and administered oxygen. They were followed by two doctors who let us know that Boaz has taken a turn for the worse and our only choice now was to take Boaz to intensive care and place him on a ventilator. We declined after calling his physician brother, as there appeared to be little, if any chance of recovery. The hospice nurse who offered home care earlier in the day never returned.

4

My sons and I spent the next few hours alone with Boaz, watching him drift in and out of sleep and holding his hand. One of his grandson's played him the violin over zoom. When we noticed that Boaz stopped breathing we notified the nurses. Soon a doctor came in hurriedly and declared him to be deceased. We were left alone with our grief and the practical needs to make funeral arrangements. There was no familiar face of a caring doctor to address our grief.

The model of hospital and institutional care does not support patient desire for continuity of care with a trusted and familiar physician (Kahana et al., 1997; Saultz & Lochner, 2005). Even for patients who have a trusted long-term physician who is affiliated with the hospital that they enter, as my husband did, treatment is taken over by teams of "hospitalist" physicians who have little prior knowledge of the patient and are not in a position to offer meaningful support as patients and their families must confront the end of life (White & Glazier 2011). This fits well with recent literature about physicians' loss of professional autonomy as they have turned into "providers" and their work has become mechanical, timed, and structured (Constand et al., 2014).

My late husband Boaz and I have written about patient preferences for end of life care (Kahana, Dan, Kahana, & Kercher, 2004). In later work we addressed potential challenges faced by older health care consumers in gaining access to quality end of life care (Kahana et al., 2014). Our lived experiences, as Boaz neared the end of life, reinforced concerns about access that we previously articulated based on research perspectives. The emotional turmoil we experienced as we faced a beloved family member's final hour were not addressed by any health care providers. We found that no one offered support to families who made the recommended choices against futile efforts toward extending life.

There were three of us, family members, in the hospital room with Boaz as he reached the end of life. All four of us are well-published PhD scholars who have studied health care. Yet we still encountered difficult problems within the system and could not achieve effective advocacy. We discovered that when faced with a health crisis like Boaz's, it's difficult to put one's research into practice—especially when there weren't any familiar nurses or doctors around to advocate for Boaz or just to explain the true nature of his condition.

There is a positive role that palliative care and hospice might play in the process of end-of-life care (Jennings et al., 2010). Unfortunately, there appears to be poor communication between teams of specialists providing traditional, intervention-oriented care and those offering comfort care in the hospital setting (Nolan & Mock, 2004). In our case, after we refused to put my husband on a ventilator, no physicians entered his room until after he passed away. Even though the hospital offered both palliative and hospice care, in practice these care options did not help us.

Having commented on our difficult bereavement experiences and our loss of a beloved elderly family member, I now turn to the solace that a new volume of the *Journal of Elder Policy* brings through the publication of creative efforts to better understand and hopefully improve elder policies.

What Our Current Issue Offers in Terms of Improving Policies for Older Adults

There are excellent insights offered about diverse components of elder policy discussed in the current issue. A number of papers touch upon treatment and health care of older adults as they near the end of life. The problems and potential of **healthcare advocacy** are considered by Gary Kreps. **Planning for retirement and future-care** are topics addressed by Silvia Sorensen and colleagues. **Elder abuse** is the topic of the paper by Georgia Anetzberger. The problems and prospects for **treatment of elderly prisoners** are discussed in the work of Tina Maschi and collaborators. **Racial differences in retirement security** are the focus of the paper by Richard Johnson. The broader societal context for **segmentation of the life course** is addressed by Dale Dannefer and his colleagues. All of these articles make important points that are relevant to older adults' life experiences.

The paper by **Gary Kreps** addresses **Health Advocacy and Health Communication for Elderly Health Care Consumers**. Kreps notes the powerful role that health advocacy can have for older adults who are navigating the health care system. He explains that health advocacy (individual or organizational) can enhance patient satisfaction, quality of care, and improve health outcomes of older adults. He outlines important communication strategies that health advocates must develop to guide older consumers through their health care decisions. Kreps' focus on health care advocacy is closely aligned with my personal observations about limitations in the delivery of end-of-life care in a hospital context. He points out that "many elderly health care consumers do not receive adequate advocacy support and have difficulty shaping health care policies and practices due to problems with ageism and power imbalances within health care systems that accord far more authority to health care providers and administrators than to consumers in the delivery of care. This limits elders' participation and influence in health care."

Georgia Anetzberger, in her article **The Elder Abuse Policy Landscape in the United States,** provides a thorough review of elder abuse related public policy in the United States. She showcases how elder abuse has evolved from being viewed as a social problem to a crime and medical syndrome. While policies have been put into place to combat elder abuse, Anetzberger points out both the important successes and shortcomings of such policies. The paper concludes with the argument that risk factors for elder abuse could be diminished if policies were in place to ensure the financial, medical, and social needs of older adults were met. Relating the concept of elder abuse to end of life experiences, one is confronted with a landscape of neglected patients often encounter close to the end of life. Explanations for interventions or for the lack thereof appear to diminish in frequency as the patient is increasingly perceived as an object of care, rather than a partner in care. Doctors and nurses often address the family member, rather than the patient, when request is made for explanations. This is what Boaz and I both experienced.

Perspectives on Aging Related Preparation (ARP) is discussed in an article prepared by **Silvia Sörensen Rachel Missell, Alexander Eustice-Corwin, and Dorine Otieno**. This article is focused on understanding both antecedents and consequences of aging related preparation (ARP) in the context of social policy. The authors differentiate planning in four different domains: retirement, housing, future care needs, and advance directives for end-of-life care. They note that even where elders consider general plans, concrete planning is rare. Many older adults disregard the possibility for increasing frailty and care needs. Advance care planning is more common, as it is mandated by the health care system. Community dwelling older adults report general plans for their future needs with no specific notion of how to implement these preferences. Only 1% to 15% report having *concrete* plans for their care (Black et al., 2008). The authors note that although advance directives are mandated, they are not well understood. This was certainly the case in Boaz's hospital experience. Major barriers to aging-related preparation include insufficient internal and external resources. Structural barriers include existing policies that inhibit meaningful care planning. The authors provide recommendations for improved goal setting as useful individual strategies coupled with more age-friendly environments that provide structural supports for effective planning.

Aging in Prison is the topic of the article by authors **Tina Maschi, Keith Morgen, Annette Hintenach, Adriana Kaye, and Karen Bullock**. They provide an in-depth overview of the global aging prison population and the issues related to this group (e.g., poor health, early mortality, risk for dementia). This article proposes a paradigm shift from a competition and conflict approach that focuses on punishment and retribution, to a caring justice partnership (CJP) model which promotes a more compassionate response. The goal of Maschi et al.'s CJP model is to "promote, facilitate, endorse, and celebrate care for one another during life's most testing moments and experiences." The authors argue that this response is more humane for those who are older, disabled, and dying in prison, and has relevance for other communities such as those suffering from homelessness or natural or human-made disasters. Although it might appear that prisoners and seriously ill hospitalized patients have little in common, it is difficult to escape the fact that hospitals share attributes characterizing total institutions and manifest congregate, segregate, and institutional control features (Goffman, 1958).

Richard Johnson's paper is concerned with **The Black-White gap in financial security during retirement**. He points to deficiencies in income protection for the poor and particularly racial minorities, who depend on Social Security primarily during their retirement years. More limited employment opportunities of younger blacks also result in financial insecurity in late life. Policy recommendations include shoring up social security and SSI payments. The author also calls for better opportunities for younger racial minorities to achieve home ownership and boost income to be better situated in their old age. Increasing minimum benefits would be desirable as this would help the neediest recipients. Additional measures that would require less financial investment by government include "ensuring that Blacks are treated fairly in credit, housing, and labor markets."

Age-Differentiated vs. Age-Integrated: Neoliberal Policy and The Future of the Life Course by authors **Dale Dannefer, Jielu Lin & George Gonos** focuses on more macro-societal phenomena. The authors provide a detailed look at the differences between the age-segmented institutionalized tripartite life course and the age-integrated alternative proposed by Matilda Riley. Their paper examines the devastating impact that neoliberal social policies (e.g., deregulation of business, privatization of public services, tax cuts, and cuts to social welfare programs) have had on the components of the life course: education, work, retirement. Their paper walks the reader through policy changes that have the potential to rebuild the institutional life course in a way that would improve individual and group well-being. These changes include policies related to universal basic income, baby bond proposals, living wage requirements, progressive tax policies, and free college education. The reforms advocated by these authors offer a promise for improved medical care at the end of life as well.

Contextualizing Essays in This Volume of *JEP* as Relevant to Policy, Practice and Elders' Lived Experiences

The articles presented in this volume of *JEP* call attention to both the depth and breadth of late life needs. While such needs require advances in policy and practice, they also entail simple notions of "common decency" in implementation of existing policies (Schorr, 1986). People who lack social capital, financial resources, and social supports face special problems in navigating challenges of ill health and navigating the health care system. Racial discrimination also puts older adults at special risk (Williams, Neighbors, & Jackson, 2003).

The healthcare and service delivery systems become particularly challenging as personal vulnerability increases close to the end of life. My hope is that offering my personal reflections about end-of-life care and needs of the bereaved in this editorial will motivate readers to critically evaluate the essays published in this volume from the vantage point of elders who experience the policy initiatives discussed. Not only do older adults benefit from policies that meet their personal and social needs, but their lived experience needs to match the stated policy goals. To the extent that policy and practice implementation is inadequate, even the most well intended policies will fall short of improving quality of late life.

During the most vulnerable phases of life, formal services alone are likely to be insufficient and older persons depend on the informal supports of family and close friends. Based on the strong emotional bonds with these individuals, the vulnerable elder can be reassured that their dignity and needs will be respected. Members of informal support networks are also more likely to be familiar with values and preferences of the frail elder and can try to meet even unarticulated needs. Consequently, the elder in need and their family members can serve as useful guides to implementation of formal services and policies. Close to the end of life it is especially important that practitioners communicate with family members and significant others, since the elder may no longer be able to advocate for themselves.

Compassionate care is the concept most closely associated with providing responsive care close to the end of life. Compassionate care is considered to involve "a relationship characterized by empathy, emotional support and efforts to understand and relieve a person's distress suffering and concerns" (Mannion, 2014, p.115). A systematic review of the literature Tehranineshat et al. (2019) found that compassionate care involves ethical and spiritual values of staff, effective communication, professional skills, and positive involvement with patients.

Healthcare environments play an important role in enabling doctors and nurses to deliver compassionate care (Christiansen et al., 2015). To understand the connection between policies to help vulnerable elders and the lived experience of service recipients, it is also important to consider perspectives, experiences, and autonomy of key health care providers (Friedberg et al., 2014). To the extent that physicians, nurses, and other health care professionals can work while maintaining professional autonomy, patients' health care experiences are likely to be improved.

Educational programs for staff have been cited as promoting compassionate care, but they appear less important than the value placed on humanistic care by health care organizations.

As I noted earlier, my late husband Boaz was an optimist who believed that scientific research and devoted teaching can improve the world, specifically the lives of older people. I conclude this essay by echoing this optimism and expressing the hope that the essays published in the *Journal of Elder Policy* can ultimately contribute to improving older adults' life experiences. As Boaz aptly put it, **"we learn from every experience and need to put our learning to good use to help others."**

Mejorar la experiencia del final de la vida de los pacientes ancianos y sus familias: La política y la práctica no llegan a brindar comodidad y apoyo

Este editorial está dedicado a mi difunto esposo Boaz Kahana y a los pacientes mayores que enfrentan el final de su vida en hospitales de cuidados intensivos.

El 6 de noviembre de 2020, perdí a mi esposo, alma gemela y colaborador de investigación de 58 años, el Dr. Boaz Kahana. Booz fue un erudito eminente, un maestro y mentor devoto y premiado, y un príncipe de hombre. Se retiró de su puesto como profesor de psicología en la Universidad Estatal de Cleveland en diciembre de 2019, menos de un año antes de su muerte. Durante su breve retiro, estaba completando un libro para estudiantes universitarios de primera generación, estudiando idiomas extranjeros y leyendo revistas científicas. Murió en uno de los principales hospitales de Estados Unidos. Tenía 86 años y era un sobreviviente a largo plazo de 21 años de la cirugía de Whipple. Luchó una valiente batalla para sobrevivir. Nuestro médico de atención primaria me llamó para darme el pésame y me dijo que mi "feroz defensa" y mi participación en la atención de Boaz probablemente le hayan extendido la vida.

Al presentar el segundo volumen del Journal of Elder Policy en medio del duelo por Boaz y el persistente trauma global de COVID 19, me gustaría aprovechar mis experiencias de vida para explorar las áreas liminales entre la vejez, la mala salud y las deficiencias. en las prácticas de atención de la salud y el apoyo social a medida que las personas se acercan al final de la vida. También mencionaré brevemente los desafíos de los ancianos en duelo. Mi principal preocupación se relaciona con las preguntas: ¿Cómo se traducen en prácticas las políticas, como las presentadas y discutidas en el Journal of Elder Policy y otras, y cómo experimentan las personas mayores y sus familias las prácticas predominantes?

Los artículos de este volumen abarcan un amplio espectro de desafíos en la vejez y soluciones políticas que podrían abordar estos desafíos. En este editorial espero relacionarlos con la experiencia vivida de acercarse al final de la vida. Me concentro en nuestra vulnerabilidad y humanidad comunes, que trascienden las cuestiones políticas específicas. Robert Binstock (1989) explicó las complejas interfaces entre las políticas públicas y la implementación. Señaló que las cadenas jerárquicas a través de las cuales se ejecutan las políticas son extensas. En relación con los programas de servicios sociales y de salud, sugirió que es el empleado de la organización de servicio quien implementa las políticas diseñadas por los formuladores de políticas y experimentadas por los clientes.

Cuando las poderosas olas de dolor me invaden, de repente las abstracciones de la investigación intelectual sobre las políticas sociales se desvanecen en un segundo plano. Son solo los recuerdos íntimos y el deseo de mejorar las experiencias de muerte y duelo de otros seres humanos lo que me levanta. Siento que es útil colocar los artículos abstractos y académicos que publicamos en un contexto humano de experiencia vivida para apreciar plenamente su relevancia y contribuciones. Mis comentarios en este editorial abarcan tanto las observaciones de los últimos días de mi esposo como mis propias experiencias al ser un anciano lidiando con la pérdida y el estatus social alterado de la viudez.

Poco después de la muerte de Booz y justo antes del Día de Acción de Gracias, experimenté un impacto cuando recibí una llamada bien intencionada de un voluntario, que estaba afiliado a una organización comunitaria local. Me dijo que, como viuda reciente, tenía derecho a una comida gratis que me podían entregar para el Día de Acción de Gracias. Si bien es bueno que exista este servicio, especialmente para los adultos mayores que pueden enfrentar problemas de seguridad alimentaria durante esta pandemia, hubo poca empatía por mi dolor en esta interacción. La atención se centró únicamente en la implementación de la prestación de servicios que reflejara una política social.

Le agradecí a la persona que llamó y le dije que no necesitaría este beneficio y colgué el teléfono con lágrimas rodando por mi rostro. En mi mente aparecieron vívidas imágenes del pasado Día de Acción de Gracias cuando Boaz y yo invitamos a nuestra casa a nuestros estudiantes nacionales e internacionales que no podían viajar a casa para las vacaciones. Recordé darles la bienvenida con un espíritu de gratitud como invitados importantes en nuestra casa participando de una comida casera en una mesa festiva. No solo perdí a mi mejor amigo y socio durante casi 60 años, sino que mi interacción con este proveedor de servicios me hizo sentir como si estuviera reducido a un caso de caridad solitario en busca de una cena de Acción de Gracias gratis.

Como académicos, abogamos por mejores políticas sociales para los ancianos, pero rara vez pensamos en lo que se siente al estar en el extremo receptor de los derechos. ¿Nuestras políticas tienen en cuenta la rica historia de vida de las personas mayores que reciben cuidados? ¿Los responsables de la formulación de políticas y los proveedores de servicios tienen en cuenta las necesidades emocionales y espirituales? ¿Cuánto respeto reciben los destinatarios del servicio?

En su libro *Being Mortal* (2014), Atul Gawande ofrece información importante sobre la desconexión entre las necesidades y aspiraciones de los adultos mayores cerca del final de sus vidas, y la comprensión de esas necesidades por parte de los proveedores de atención médica. Durante las últimas estancias de los pacientes en un hospital o un hogar de ancianos, donde la mayoría de los ancianos mueren, hay poca comunicación sobre los temores, las opciones y los deseos de los pacientes. Nuestras políticas han evolucionado para solicitar directivas anticipadas a los pacientes, pero hacemos poco para asegurarnos de que comprendan completamente las implicaciones de dichas directivas.

En el caso de mi esposo, un médico de cuidados paliativos bien intencionado pasó por su habitación poco después de su llegada al hospital. El médico conversó sobre las revistas científicas que estaba leyendo mi esposo. Casi como una ocurrencia tardía, le preguntó a mi esposo si, "en el improbable caso de que su salud empeorara aún más, ¿todavía querría intervenciones para extender su vida?" El eterno optimista, Boaz respondió: "Por supuesto, me gustaría obtener toda la ayuda que pudiera obtener". El médico no explicó la naturaleza de las intervenciones al final de la vida que tenía en mente, ni la probabilidad de que tuvieran éxito. Cuando llegó el momento de tomar las decisiones finales, mis hijos y yo optamos por medidas heroicas para prolongar la vida de Boaz. Muchos médicos no explican que las medidas heroicas pueden prolongar la vida, pero no siempre brindan calidad de vida durante el tiempo que se mantiene con vida a la persona.

Boaz fue hospitalizado por recomendación de nuestro competente y atento médico de atención primaria para tratar de averiguar qué estaba causando la extrema fatiga y debilidad que había estado experimentando durante meses. Murió en el hospital 10 días después. Fue bueno que durante las últimas horas de Boaz, nuestros hijos y yo pudiéramos estar con él. Hasta ese momento, solo yo había podido visitar. Durante la pandemia, se redujo el contacto significativo de los pacientes hospitalizados y sus familiares. El hospital donde Boaz era un paciente solo permitió la visita de un miembro designado de la familia debido a preocupaciones comprensibles sobre la propagación del COVID-19.

Mi experiencia personal con una crisis al final de la vida de mi esposo y la forma en que funciona el sistema de servicios hospitalarios no es exclusiva de mí. Muchas familias durante el año pasado han experimentado de cerca el funcionamiento del sistema de atención médica durante COVID-19. Ellos también se han enfrentado a la toma de decisiones al final de la vida dentro de un sistema que tiene como objetivo armonizar los servicios, pero a menudo no da en el blanco, ya que las estructuras burocráticas y las políticas de servicio les impiden alcanzar los objetivos del cuidado compasivo (Youngson 2011; Kneafsey et al. 2016).

Mientras abogamos por mejores políticas sociales para proteger a los ancianos, los expertos generalmente se basan en la lógica y los resultados de estudios anteriores. La calidad de la atención médica rara vez se ve a través de los ojos del paciente (Gerteis 1993). Además, aunque existen estudios cualitativos para las experiencias de los pacientes, no parece que estos estudios se utilicen como evidencia para el desarrollo de políticas, ya sea porque se basan en experiencias "subjetivas" o en pequeñas muestras de estudios. En cierto sentido, no se consideran una investigación rigurosa, a pesar de que brindan una ventana a lo que es estar en el extremo receptor de las prácticas y políticas de salud. En el clima actual de prestación de servicios de salud, las consideraciones financieras y los protocolos de financiación juegan un papel importante. Estos algoritmos en evolución proporcionan pocos incentivos o incluso espacio para la atención centrada en el paciente (Constrand et al. 2014).

La atención médica tiene cada vez menos que ver con el cuidado de los pacientes y más con la prestación eficiente de servicios con el paciente, considerado como el objeto de la prestación de cuidados, más que como un ser humano que sufre (Salamon 2008; Sweet 2013). Una persona acostada en una cama incómoda, conectada a una vía intravenosa, incapaz de comer y demasiado débil para usar un baño normal, se reduce a ser un receptor pasivo de cuidados. Los pacientes gravemente enfermos no están en condiciones de hacer preguntas y expresar sus temores de abandono cuando no hay familiares presentes. Ayudar a mantener la dignidad humana y la comodidad del paciente, como cepillarse los dientes y tener una apariencia bien arreglada, no parece ser una prioridad en la lista de tareas ocupadas de los proveedores de atención (Henderson et al. 2009). Además de estar hambriento y débil, Booz también sentía frío, especialmente de noche. Le traje suéteres, guantes y un gorro, para que estuviera más cómodo. Era mi tarea, antes de irme por la noche, ayudarlo a ponerse la ropa de abrigo. Me pregunté sobre la precaria situación de otros pacientes ancianos solitarios hospitalizados sin acceso a familiares. Los médicos y enfermeras rara vez están dispuestos o son capaces de hablar sobre los temores, las preocupaciones y la comodidad de los pacientes.

Boaz se había sometido a un procedimiento exitoso para colocar un stent pancreático durante el tercer día después de su hospitalización y nos sentimos optimistas sobre su recuperación. Esta impresión se vio reforzada por el comportamiento del médico. Sin embargo, se encontró con complicaciones cuando intentaron durante cinco días establecer un régimen de nutrición artificial. No se le proporcionó comida por vía oral durante este período. Estaba claramente angustiado, incómodo y cada vez más agitado. Me susurró con temor: ¿Hasta cuándo me matarán de hambre? No tenía respuestas para él. Solo podía ofrecerme a consultar con sus enfermeras y médicos. De hecho, los médicos visitaron a Boaz en equipos de 4 o 5 especialistas a la vez. En gran medida conferenciaron entre ellos y diferentes equipos de nutrición (alimentación intravenosa frente a alimentación por sonda), y parecían preferir sus estrategias específicas. Los médicos que lo visitaron dieron pocos indicios de las perspectivas de Boaz. No se dirigieron a él directamente y nadie preguntó por el malestar que estaba experimentando.

Boaz conservó su agudeza mental hasta sus momentos finales. Como se debilitó demasiado para hablar, le di papel y bolígrafo para que pudiera escribir lo que quería. Me pedía que pusiera su reloj en la hora correcta, incluido el día. Quería la dignidad de estar orientado al tiempo. Escribió "jueves", el día antes de morir. Me estaba recordando en qué día de la semana poner su reloj. Esto me hace pensar en la importancia de proteger y garantizar la dignidad, cerca del final de la vida.

El jueves por la noche no hubo indicios de que la condición de Booz empeorara. Llegué el viernes por la mañana sorprendida al encontrar a varios miembros del personal rodeándolo. Me dijeron que esperara afuera mientras intentaban succionar una pastilla que Booz aspiró. Mi impresión fue que lo habían logrado y no me informaron que su condición se volviera crítica. Un representante de Hospice vino más tarde el viernes por la mañana y me preguntó si me gustaría llevar a Boaz a casa para que pudiera recibir cuidados reconfortantes y pasar tiempo rodeado de su familia. Una vez más, no se mencionó su inminente desaparición y no le pregunté cuánto tiempo tenía. Acepté con entusiasmo la idea de traerlo a casa. Como ahora se le consideraba un paciente de cuidados paliativos, nuestros hijos pudieron visitarlo. Ambos llegaron rápidamente.

A primera hora de la tarde, vino un fisioterapeuta e hizo algunas maniobras en el cuerpo de Boaz. Durante este proceso, la respiración de Boaz se dificultó. Las enfermeras entraron rápidamente y le administraron oxígeno. Fueron seguidos por dos médicos que nos informaron que Boaz había empeorado y nuestra única opción ahora era llevarlo a cuidados intensivos y colocarlo en un ventilador. Nos negamos después de llamar a su hermano médico, ya que parecía haber poca o ninguna posibilidad de recuperación. La enfermera del hospicio que ofreció atención domiciliaria más temprano ese día nunca regresó.

Mis hijos y yo pasamos las siguientes horas solos con Boaz, viéndolo entrar y salir del sueño y tomar su mano. Uno de sus nietos le tocó el violín por Zoom. Cuando notamos que Boaz dejó de respirar, notificamos a las enfermeras. Pronto, un médico entró apresuradamente y lo declaró fallecido. Nos quedamos solos con nuestro dolor y las necesidades prácticas para hacer los arreglos del funeral. No había un rostro familiar de un médico que se preocupara por nuestro dolor.

El modelo de atención hospitalaria e institucional no respalda el deseo del paciente de continuar la atención con un médico familiar y de confianza (Saultz & Lochner 2005, Kahana et al. 1997). Incluso para los pacientes que tienen un médico de confianza a largo plazo que está afiliado al hospital al que ingresan, como lo hizo mi esposo, el tratamiento está a cargo de equipos de médicos "hospitalistas" que tienen poco conocimiento previo del paciente y no están en posición para ofrecer un apoyo significativo cuando los pacientes y sus familias deben afrontar el final de la vida (White & Glazier 2011). Esto encaja bien con la literatura reciente sobre la pérdida de autonomía profesional de los médicos a medida que se han convertido en "proveedores" y su trabajo se ha vuelto mecánico, cronometrado y estructurado (Constand et al. 2014).

Mi difunto esposo Boaz y yo hemos escrito sobre las preferencias de los pacientes para la atención al final de la vida (Kahana, Dan, Kahana & Kercher 2004). En un trabajo posterior abordamos los posibles desafíos que enfrentan los consumidores de atención médica de edad avanzada para obtener acceso a una atención de calidad al final de la vida (E. Kahana et al. 2014). Nuestras experiencias vividas, a medida que Booz se acercaba al final de la vida, reforzaron las preocupaciones sobre el acceso que articulamos anteriormente con base en perspectivas de investigación. Los proveedores de atención médica no abordaron la confusión emocional que experimentamos al enfrentarnos a la última hora de un familiar querido.

Descubrimos que nadie ofreció apoyo a las familias que tomaron las decisiones recomendadas contra los esfuerzos inútiles para prolongar la vida.

Éramos tres, miembros de la familia, en la habitación del hospital con Boaz cuando llegó al final de su vida. Los cuatro somos académicos de doctorado bien publicados que hemos estudiado el cuidado de la salud. Sin embargo, todavía nos encontramos con problemas difíciles dentro del sistema y no pudimos lograr una promoción eficaz. Descubrimos que cuando nos enfrentamos a una crisis de salud como la de Boaz, es difícil poner en práctica la investigación de uno, especialmente cuando no había enfermeras o médicos familiares que defendieran a Boaz o simplemente explicaran la verdadera naturaleza de su condición.

Los cuidados paliativos y los cuidados paliativos pueden desempeñar un papel positivo en el proceso de cuidados al final de la vida (Jennings et al. 2010). Desafortunadamente, parece haber una mala comunicación entre los equipos de especialistas que brindan atención tradicional orientada a la intervención y los que ofrecen atención de confort en el ámbito hospitalario (Nolan y Mock 2004). En nuestro caso, después de que nos negamos a poner a mi esposo en un ventilador, ningún médico entró a su habitación hasta después de su muerte. Aunque el hospital ofrecía cuidados paliativos y de cuidados paliativos, en la práctica estas opciones de atención no nos ayudaron.

Habiendo comentado nuestras difíciles experiencias de duelo y la pérdida de un querido miembro anciano de la familia, ahora me refiero al consuelo que brinda un nuevo volumen del Journal of Elder Policy a través de la publicación de esfuerzos creativos para comprender mejor y, con suerte, mejorar las políticas sobre ancianos.

Lo que ofrece nuestro número actual en términos de mejorar las políticas para los adultos mayores

Se ofrecen ideas excelentes sobre los diversos componentes de la política de personas mayores que se analizan en el número actual. Varios artículos abordan el tratamiento y la atención médica de los adultos mayores a medida que se acercan al final de la vida. Gary Kreps considera los problemas y el potencial de la promoción de la salud. La planificación para la jubilación y el cuidado futuro son temas abordados por Silvia Sorensen y sus colegas. El abuso de ancianos es el tema del artículo de Georgia Anetzberger. Los problemas y perspectivas de tratamiento de los presos ancianos se discuten en el trabajo de Tina Maschi y colaboradores. Las diferencias raciales en la seguridad de la jubilación son el tema central del artículo de Richard Johnson. Dale Dannefer y sus colegas abordan el contexto social más amplio para la segmentación del curso de la vida. Todos estos artículos destacan puntos importantes que son relevantes para las experiencias de vida de los adultos mayores.

El document de **Gary Kreps** tiene le título de **Health Advocacy and Health Communication for Elderly Health Care Consumers**. Kreps señala el poderoso papel que puede tener la defensa de la salud para los adultos mayores que navegan por el sistema de atención médica. Explica que la defensa de la salud (individual u organizativa) puede mejorar la satisfacción del paciente, la calidad de la atención y mejorar los resultados de salud de los adultos mayores. Él describe importantes estrategias de comunicación que los defensores de la salud deben desarrollar para guiar a los consumidores mayores a través de sus decisiones de atención médica. El enfoque de Kreps en la defensa de la atención médica está estrechamente alineado con mis observaciones personales sobre las limitaciones en la prestación de atención al final de la vida en un contexto hospitalario. Señala que "muchos consumidores de atención médica de edad avanzada no reciben el apoyo de defensa adecuado y tienen dificultades para dar forma a las políticas y prácticas de atención médica debido a problemas de discriminación por edad y desequilibrios de poder dentro de los sistemas de atención médica que otorgan mucha más autoridad a los proveedores y administradores de atención médica que a consumidores en la prestación de cuidados. Esto limita la participación e influencia de los ancianos en la atención médica".

Georgia Anetzberger, en su artículo, **The Elder Abuse Policy Landscape in the United States,** proporciona una revisión completa de la política pública relacionada con el abuso de personas mayores en los Estados Unidos. Ella muestra cómo el abuso de personas mayores ha evolucionado de ser visto como un problema social a un crimen y un síndrome médico. Si bien se han implementado políticas para combatir el abuso de personas mayores, Anetzberger señala tanto los importantes éxitos como las deficiencias de tales políticas. El documento concluye con el argumento de que los factores de riesgo de abuso de personas mayores podrían reducirse si se implementaran políticas para garantizar que se satisfagan las necesidades financieras, médicas y sociales de las personas mayores. Al relacionar el concepto de abuso de ancianos con las experiencias del final de la vida, uno se enfrenta a un panorama de pacientes abandonados que a menudo se encuentran cerca del final de la vida. Las explicaciones de las intervenciones o de la falta de ellas parecen disminuir en frecuencia a medida que el paciente se percibe cada vez más como un objeto de atención, más que como un socio en la atención. Los médicos y enfermeras a menudo se dirigen al miembro de la familia, en lugar del paciente, cuando se solicita explicaciones. Esto es lo que experimentamos Boaz y yo.

Perspectives on Aging Related Preparation (ARP) es el tíctulo del artículo de **Silvia Sörensen Rachel Missell, Alexander Eustice-Corwin y Dorine Otieno**. Este artículo se centra en comprender tanto los antecedentes como las consecuencias de la preparación relacionada con el envejecimiento (ARP) en el contexto de la política social. Los autores diferencian la planificación en cuatro dominios diferentes: jubilación, vivienda, necesidades de atención futura y directivas anticipadas para la atención al final de la vida. Señalan que incluso cuando los ancianos consideran planes generales, la planificación concreta es rara. Muchos adultos mayores ignoran la posibilidad de aumentar la fragilidad y las necesidades de atención. La planificación anticipada de la atención es más común, ya que es un mandato del sistema de atención médica. Los adultos mayores que viven en la comunidad informan planes generales para sus necesidades futuras sin una noción específica de cómo implementar estas preferencias. Solo del 1% al 15% informa tener planes concretos para su atención (Black et al. 2008). Los autores señalan que aunque las instrucciones anticipadas son obligatorias, no se comprenden bien. Este fue ciertamente el caso de la experiencia hospitalaria de Boaz. Las principales barreras para la preparación relacionada con el envejecimiento incluyen recursos internos y externos insuficientes. Las barreras estructurales incluyen políticas existentes que inhiben una planificación significativa de la atención. Los autores brindan recomendaciones para mejorar el establecimiento de metas como estrategias individuales útiles junto con entornos más amigables con las personas mayores que brindan apoyo estructural para una planificación efectiva.

Aging in Prison es el tema del documento de **Tina Maschi, Keith Morgen, Annette Hintenach, Adriana Kaye, y Karen Bullock**. Proporcionan una visión general en profundidad del envejecimiento de la población carcelaria mundial y los problemas relacionados con este grupo (por ejemplo, mala salud, mortalidad temprana, riesgo de demencia). Este artículo propone un cambio de paradigma desde un enfoque de competencia y conflicto que se centra en el castigo y la retribución, a un modelo de asociación de justicia solidaria (CJP) que promueve una respuesta más compasiva. El objetivo del modelo CJP de Maschi et al. Es "promover, facilitar, respaldar y celebrar el cuidado mutuo durante los momentos y experiencias más difíciles de la vida". Los autores argumentan que esta respuesta es más humana para las personas mayores, discapacitadas y que mueren en prisión, y tiene relevancia para otras comunidades, como las que sufren de falta de vivienda o desastres naturales o provocados por el hombre. Aunque pueda parecer que los prisioneros y los pacientes hospitalizados gravemente enfermos tienen poco en común, es difícil escapar al hecho de que los hospitales comparten atributos que caracterizan a las instituciones totales y manifiestan características de control institucional, de congregación y segregación (Goffman, 1958).

Richard Johnson escribe sobre el siguiente tema: **The Black-White gap in financial security during retirement**. Señala las deficiencias en la protección de los ingresos para los pobres y, en particular, las minorías raciales, que dependen del Seguro Social principalmente durante sus años de jubilación. Las oportunidades de empleo más limitadas de los negros más jóvenes también resultan en inseguridad financiera en la vejez. Las recomendaciones de política incluyen apuntalar los pagos de seguridad social y SSI. El autor también pide mejores oportunidades para que las minorías raciales más jóvenes logren la propiedad de una vivienda y aumenten los ingresos para que estén mejor situadas en su vejez. Sería deseable aumentar los beneficios mínimos, ya que esto ayudaría a los beneficiarios más necesitados. Las medidas adicionales que requerirían una menor inversión financiera por parte del gobierno incluyen "garantizar que los negros sean tratados de manera justa en el crédito, la vivienda y los mercados laborales".

Age-Differentiated vs. Age-Integrated: Neoliberal Policy and The Future of the Life Course de los autores: **Dale Dannefer, Jielu Lin y George Gonos** se centra en fenómenos más macrosociales. Los autores ofrecen una mirada detallada a las diferencias entre el curso de vida tripartito institucionalizado segmentado por edad y la alternativa integrada por edad propuesta por Matilda Riley. Su artículo examina el impacto devastador que las políticas sociales neoliberales (por ejemplo, desregulación de empresas, privatización de servicios públicos, recortes de impuestos y recortes a programas de bienestar social) han tenido en los componentes del curso de la vida: educación, trabajo, jubilación. Su artículo guía al lector a través de cambios de política que tienen el potencial de reconstruir el curso de la vida institucional de una manera que mejoraría el bienestar individual y grupal. Estos cambios incluyen políticas relacionadas con el ingreso básico universal, propuestas de bonos para bebés, requisitos de salario digno, políticas de impuestos progresivos y educación universitaria gratuita. Las reformas defendidas por estos autores también prometen mejorar la atención médica al final de la vida.

Contextualización de los ensayos de este volumen de *JEP* como relevantes para la política, la práctica y las experiencias vividas por los adultos mayores

Los artículos presentados en este volumen de *JEP* llaman la atención sobre la profundidad y amplitud de las necesidades de la vejez. Si bien tales necesidades requieren avances en las políticas y la práctica, también implican nociones simples de "decencia común" en la implementación de las políticas existentes (Schorr 1986). Las personas que carecen de capital social, recursos financieros y apoyo social enfrentan problemas especiales para enfrentar los desafíos de la mala salud y navegar por el sistema de atención médica. La discriminación racial también pone a los adultos mayores en riesgo especial (Williams, Neighbours & Jackson 2003).

Los sistemas de prestación de servicios y atención médica se vuelven particularmente desafiantes a medida que la vulnerabilidad personal aumenta cerca del final de la vida. Mi esperanza es que ofrecer mis reflexiones personales sobre el cuidado al final de la vida y las necesidades de los deudos en este editorial motive a los lectores a evaluar críticamente los ensayos publicados en este volumen desde el punto de vista de los ancianos que experimentan las iniciativas políticas discutidas. Los adultos mayores no solo se benefician de las políticas que satisfacen sus necesidades personales y sociales, sino que su experiencia de vida debe coincidir con los objetivos establecidos de la política. En la medida en que la implementación de políticas y prácticas sea inadecuada, incluso las políticas mejor intencionadas no lograrán mejorar la calidad de la vida en la vejez.

Durante las fases más vulnerables de la vida, es probable que los servicios formales por sí solos sean insuficientes y las personas mayores dependan del apoyo informal de familiares y amigos cercanos. Sobre la base de los fuertes lazos emocionales con estas personas, el anciano vulnerable puede estar seguro de que se respetarán su dignidad y necesidades. Los miembros de las redes de apoyo informales también tienen más probabilidades de estar familiarizados con los valores y preferencias del anciano frágil y pueden tratar de satisfacer incluso las necesidades no articuladas. En consecuencia, los ancianos necesitados y sus familiares pueden servir como guías útiles para la implementación de políticas y servicios formales. Cerca del final de la vida, es especialmente importante que los profesionales se comuniquen con los miembros de la familia y otras personas importantes, ya que es posible que el anciano ya no pueda defenderse por sí mismo.

La atención compasiva es el concepto más estrechamente asociado con la prestación de atención receptiva cerca del final de la vida. Se considera que el cuidado compasivo implica "una relación caracterizada por la empatía, el apoyo emocional y los esfuerzos por comprender y aliviar el sufrimiento y las preocupaciones de una persona" (Mannion 2014, p.115). Una revisión sistemática de la literatura Tehranineshat et al. (2019) encontraron que el cuidado compasivo involucra valores éticos y espirituales del personal, comunicación efectiva, habilidades profesionales y participación positiva con los pacientes.

Los entornos de atención médica desempeñan un papel importante al permitir que los médicos y enfermeras brinden una atención compasiva (Christiansen et al. 2015). Para comprender la conexión entre las políticas para ayudar a los ancianos vulnerables y la experiencia vivida por los destinatarios del servicio, también es importante considerar las perspectivas, las experiencias y la autonomía de los proveedores de atención médica clave (Friedberg et al. 2014). En la medida en que los médicos, enfermeras y otros profesionales de la salud puedan trabajar manteniendo la autonomía profesional, es probable que mejoren las experiencias de atención médica de los pacientes.

Se ha citado que los programas educativos para el personal promueven la atención compasiva, pero parecen menos importantes que el valor que las organizaciones de atención de la salud atribuyen a la atención humanística.

Como señalé anteriormente, mi difunto esposo Boaz era un optimista que creía que la investigación científica y la enseñanza dedicada pueden mejorar el mundo, específicamente las vidas de las personas mayores. Concluyo este ensayo haciéndome eco de este optimismo y expresando la esperanza de que los ensayos publicados en el Journal of Elder Policy puedan contribuir en última instancia a mejorar las experiencias de vida de los adultos mayores. Como bien dijo Boaz, **"Aprendemos de cada experiencia y debemos hacer un buen uso de nuestro aprendizaje para ayudar a los demás".**

改善老年病人及其家庭的临终经历：
政策和实践无法充分提供舒适和支持

> 本篇社论献给我的已故丈夫*Boaz Kahana*和在急诊医院面临生命终点的其他老年病人。

2020年11月6日，我失去了我的丈夫兼灵魂伴侣、共事58年的研究合作者，Boaz Kahana博士。Boaz是一名杰出学者、一名获奖的敬业教师及导师、还是一个杰出的男人。他是克利夫兰州立大学的心理学教授，于2019年12月退休，退休不满一年便去世。在他的短暂退休生活中，他为第一代大学生创作一本书、学习外语并阅读科学杂志。他在美国最著名的一所医院里去世。他享年86岁，并且在胰十二指肠切除术后幸存了21年。他顽强地抗击病魔。我们的初级保健医生打电话给我表示悼念，并告诉我，我的"强烈倡导"和对Boaz的悉心照顾很有可能延长了他的生命。

在我为Boaz感到悲痛和在全球新冠肺炎（COVID-19）疫情期间介绍《老年政策期刊》第二卷时，我想用自己的生活经历探究当人们接近生命终点时，老龄、生病、医疗实践缺乏以及社会支持之间的过渡区域。我也将简要提及丧失亲友的老年人所面临的挑战。我的主要顾虑与下列疑问相关：像《老年政策期刊》和其他期刊中所呈现和探讨的政策如何转化为实践，并且老年人及其家庭是如何经历主流实践的？

本卷收录的文章包括一系列广泛的晚年生活挑战和可能应对这些挑战的政策解决措施。我希望在这篇社论中将这些挑战和措施与临终生命经历相联系。我聚焦于共同的脆弱性和人性，它们穿越特定政策议题的限制。学者Robert Binstock （1989）解释了公共政策及其执行之间的复杂关系。他指出，政策执行通过阶级链完成，这种阶级链是广泛的。至于卫生和社会服务计划，他暗示，执行政策的是服务组织的员工，而政策由决策者设计并对客户产生影响。

当我沉浸在强烈的悲痛中时，关于社会政策疑问的抽象概念突然变得不再那么重要。让我振奋起来的只有亲密的回忆和关于改善其他人的死亡经历及丧失亲友的经历的愿望。我认为，将我们发表的抽象学术文章置于人类生活经历背景中，有助于充分理解其相关性和贡献。我在本篇社论中所作的评论包含了我对丈夫临终前的观察和我作为一名应对亲人逝世和改变的丧偶社会地位的老年人的个人经历。

Boaz去世不久后，感恩节之前，我接到了一个让我震惊的善意电话，打电话的是地方社区组织的一名志愿者。她告诉我，作为一名新寡妇，我有资格在感恩节享受一顿免费外卖用餐。尽管这项服务是善意的，尤其对那些在大流行期间可能面临粮食安全危机的老年人，但这通电话并没有为我的伤痛带来共情。电话的重点仅仅是执行一项反映社会政策的服务交付。

我对她表示感谢，并告诉她我将不需要这份服务，挂断电话后我的眼泪流了下来。我的脑海中闪过了以往感恩节的生动画面，那时Boaz和我邀请无法回家过节的本土学生及国际学生到我们家。我记得以感恩的心情欢迎他们到我家做客，一起在节日餐桌上享用自制食物。我不仅仅失去了最好的朋友和近60年的伴侣，并且我与这名服务提供者的通话让我感觉我仅仅是一个孤独的、寻找免费感恩节晚餐的慈善案例。

作为学者，Boaz和我为老年人倡导更好的社会政策，但很少思考过获得方的感受。我们的政策考虑了老年护理获得者的丰富生活历史吗？决策者和服务提供商考虑了老年人的情感和精神需求吗？服务获得者得到了多少尊重？

在他的著作《最好的告别》（*Being Mortal*）（2014）中，Atul Gawande给出了重要见解，这些见解有关于老年人临终前的需求和愿望，与医疗提供者对这些需求的理解之间的断裂。大多数老年人在医院或疗养院去世，但在病人的弥留之际却几乎没有关于病人的担忧、选择和愿望的沟通。我们的政策已发展为能从病人处征求预先指示，但我们却几乎没有保证他们完全理解这些指示的意义。

以我的丈夫为例，一名善意的姑息治疗医生在他住院不久后短暂拜访了他的病房。医生和我丈夫就他正在阅读的科学杂志作了交流。几乎是一个事后思考，他问我的丈夫如果"在不太可能的情况下他的健康状况恶化，他是否还希望通过干预手段来延长生命？"Boaz这个永远的乐观主义者回答道："当然，我希望获得一切我能得到的帮助。"这名医生并没有解释临终干预措施的性质，也没有解释这些干预手段的成功率。当是时候做最终决定时，我的两个儿子和我选择不采取延长Boaz生命的干预手段。许多医生不会解释的是，这些英勇的措施可能会延长生命，但却不能保证生命延长期间病人的生命质量。

在我们称职的、关爱的初级保健医生的建议下，Boaz进入医院治疗，以期试图发现几个月来他极度疲倦和虚弱的原因。住院10天后他去世了。Boaz去世前的几个小时里，我们的儿子和我获许陪着他，这是好事。在这之前，只有我能陪着他。大流行期间，住院病人和家人的重要接触减少了。出于有关新冠肺炎的顾虑（这是可理解的），Boaz所在的医院仅允许一名家庭成员拜访病人。

我在面临丈夫死亡危机时的经历，以及医院服务系统的运作方式并不是特有的。过去一年里，许多家庭都详细经历了新冠肺炎期间医疗系统的运作。他们也在一个致力协调各项服务的系统中面临生死决策，但这个系统经常未实现目标，因为官僚结构和服务政策阻止这些服务实现人文关怀（compassionate care）的目标（Youngson 2011; Kneafsey et al. 2016）。

当我们倡导通过更好的社会政策保护老年人时，专家常常依靠以往研究的逻辑和结果。几乎没有以病人的视角看待医疗质量（Gerteis　1993）。此外，尽管存在有关病人经历的定性研究，但似乎这些研究并未被用作发展政策的依据—无论这是否归因于这些研究基于"主观"经历或研究样本量小。从某种意义上讲，它们不被视为严谨的研究，尽管其提供了一扇窗了解医疗实践和卫生政策接收方的感受。在当前医疗交付环境下，财政考量和资金协定发挥了重要作用。这些不断发展的规则几乎没有为以病人为中心的护理提供激励，甚至是空间（Constrand et al. 2014）。

医疗越来越与照顾病人不相关，而与高效服务交付相关，其中病人被视为护理交付的客体，而不是一个受难的人（Salamon 2008; Sweet 2013）。躺在不舒适的病床上、连接静脉注射、无法进食、太虚弱以至于无法使用常规卫生间，这样的病人被限制为一个被动的护理接受者。当家人不在场时，重症病人无法提问并阐明他们对被抛弃的恐惧。帮助维持病人的尊严和舒适，例如刷牙和打理好的仪容，似乎并不是护理提供者要做之事的重点（Henderson et al. 2009）。除了饥饿和虚弱，Boaz还感到寒冷，尤其在夜间。我给他带去了毛衣、手套和一顶帽子，让他感到更舒适。晚上离开医院前，帮他穿上暖和的衣服成了我的任务。我想知道其他孤独老年病人在没有家人陪伴下住院时的危险处境。医生和护士很少乐意或能够讨论病人的恐惧、担忧和舒适。

Boaz在入院第三天时成功完成了胰管支架置入手术，我们对他的康复感到乐观。内科医生的态度也加深了这种乐观印象。然而，在尝试通过人工营养进食的第五天时引起了并发症。在此期间他没有通过嘴进食。他十分沮丧、难受并越来越不安。他害怕地低声告诉我：他们还要让我饿多久？我没有回答。我只能和他的护士和医生确认这一情况。的确，每次都是四五个专家医生一起拜访Boaz。大部分时间他们与不同营养小组（静脉营养vs.灌食）交流，并且似乎都偏好各自的方案。医生几乎没有给出关于Boaz情况的信息。他们没有直接和Boaz沟通，也没有一个人询问他正在经历的不适。

Boaz在临终前一直保持着敏锐的精神状况。当他变得太虚弱以至于无法说话时，我给了他纸和笔，让他写下他的愿望。他让我将他的手表调到正确的时间，包括当天是哪一天。他想要时间准确的自尊。在他去世的前一天，他写下了"星期四"。他提醒我把手表调到准确的某一天。这让我想到保护和确保临终自尊的重要性。

星期四晚没有迹象表明Boaz的情况出现恶化。星期五早晨，我来到医院时惊讶地发现不同员工围绕着他。在他们试图从Boaz体内抽吸出一颗药丸时，我被告知在病房外等候。我的印象是，他们成功吸出了药丸，并且我没有被告知Boaz的情况变得危急。当天早上一名临终安养院的代表也随后赶来，并告诉我是否愿意将Boaz带回家进行舒适护理，并和家人共度时光。又一次，没有任何关于他即将死亡的告知，我也没有问医生他还能活多久。我激动地将他带回了家。既然他那时被视为一名临终安养病人，我们的儿子被允许拜访他。他们立即赶来了。

当天午后，一名物理治疗师过来对Boaz的身体进行了一些操作。在操作过程中，Boaz的呼吸变得吃力。护士冲了进来并进行输氧。两名医生随后赶来，告诉我们Boaz的情况出现恶化，并且我们唯一的选择是将Boaz带回重症监护室，并安上呼吸机。在我们打电话给Boaz的兄弟（一名内科医生）后，我们拒绝了请求，因为恢复的希望渺茫。早上提出提供家庭护理的临终安养院护士再也没有返回。

我和我的儿子在接下来的几小时里独自陪着Boaz，看着他时醒时睡，并握住他的手。他的一个外孙通过Zoom给他演奏了小提琴。当我们察觉Boaz停止呼吸时便通知了护士。一名医生很快赶来并宣布死亡消息。我们独自应对悲痛和有关葬礼安排的实际需求。没有一名熟悉的护理医生来关心我们的悲痛。

医院和制度护理的模式并不支持病人对由信赖的、熟悉的内科医生给与持续护理的渴望（Saultz & Lochner 2005, Kahana et al. 1997）。甚至对那些拥有一名长期可信赖的、隶属于同一医院的内科医生的病人，例如我的丈夫，治疗也被"医院医生"团队接管，他们对病人的情况知之甚少，并且当病人及其家庭必须面对死亡时他们也无法提供重要支持（White & Glazier 2011）。这符合近期文献所研究的内容，后者研究了当内科医生转变为"提供者"并且其工作变得机械、时间固定、结构化时，他们所失去的专业自主权。

我的已故丈夫Boaz与我研究过病人对临终护理的偏好（Kahana, Dan, Kahana & Kercher 2004）。之后的研究中我们研究了老年医疗消费者在获取高质量临终护理时遭遇的潜在挑战（E. Kahana et al. 2014）。随着Boaz走向生命终点，我们的生活经历加强了之前我们基于研究视角阐明的、与护理获取相关的顾虑。我们在至爱的家庭成员临终前几个小时里所经历的情感焦虑并没有得到任何医疗提供者的关注。我们发现，没有人对作出推荐选择（即反对延长生命的徒劳尝试）的家庭提供支持。

Boaz去世时，我们三个家庭成员在病房陪着他。我们四个人都是著作等身的、研究过医疗的博士学者。然而，我们仍然面临医疗系统中的困难问题，并且未能实现有效倡导。我们发现，当面临一场像Boaz这样的卫生危机时，将一个人的研究投入实践是困难的—尤其当没有任何一个熟悉的护士或医生在身旁支持Boaz或仅仅是解释他病况的真实性质。

姑息治疗和临终关怀可能在临终护理过程中发挥一个积极作用（Jennings et al. 2010）。不幸的是，提供传统的、以干预为导向的护理的专家团队，和提供医院舒适护理的专家团队之间的沟通似乎并不充分（Nolan & Mock 2004）。以我们为例，在我们拒绝对Boaz使用呼吸机时，没有一名内科医生在他去世前走进过他的病房。尽管这家医院提供姑息治疗和临终护理，但在实践中这些护理选项并没有为我们提供帮助。

在对丧失亲人的艰难经历和至爱的老年家庭成员的去世加以评论后，我现在稍感安慰，因为新一卷的《老年政策期刊》通过发表创造性文章来更好的理解老年政策，并希望能改善老年政策。

本期内容在改进老年人政策方面提供了什么

本期内容探讨了就老年政策的不同部分所提出的精彩见解。一些文章提及了老年人临终时的治疗和医疗。学者Gary Kreps衡量了医疗倡导（**health-care advocacy**）的问题和潜能。学者Silvia Sorensen等人研究了退休规划和未来-护理。学者Georgia Anetzberger的文章主题是虐待老年人。学者Tina Maschi等人的文章探讨了针对老年囚犯治疗的问题和前景。学者Richard Johnson的文章重点是退休保障中的种族差异。学者Dale Dannefer等人研究了有关生命历程分区的更广的社会背景。所有这些文章都作出了与老年人的生活经历相关的重要见解。

Gary Kreps的文章研究了针对老年医疗消费者的卫生倡导和卫生传播。Kreps指出了卫生倡导能对正在摸索医疗系统的老年人产生的重要作用。他解释道，卫生倡导（个人或组织）能提升病人的满意度、护理质量，并改善老年人的卫生结果。他概述了卫生倡导者必须发展的重要传播战略，以期指导老年消费者作出医疗决策。Kreps对医疗倡导的关注与我在医院临终护理交付限制方面的个人观察密切一致。他指出，"许多老年医疗消费者没有获得足够的倡导支持，并因医疗系统内的年龄歧视和权力不平衡等问题而在影响医疗政策及实践一事上遭遇困难，这样的医疗系统在护理交付过程中将更多权力交给医疗提供商和管理者，而不是消费者。此举限制了老年人在医疗中的参与和影响。"

Georgia Anetzberger在其文章《关于虐待老年人的美国政策概况》中全面审视了与虐待老年人相关的美国公共政策。她展示了虐待老年人一事如何从被视为一个社会问题发展为犯罪和医学综合征。尽管存在相关政策打击老年人虐待，但Anetzberger指出了这类政策的重要成果和缺陷。这篇文章的结论主张，老年人虐待的风险因素能减少，如果存在相应政策确保满足老年人的财务、医疗和社会需求。将老年人虐待的概念与死亡经历相联系，个体面临的是病人在临终前经常被忽视的场景。当病人越来越被视为一个护理客体、而不是需要护理的人时，有关干预或干预不足的解释的频率似乎会减少。当寻求病情解释时，医生和护士经常与家庭成员交流，而不是与病人沟通。Boaz和我都经历了这一情况。

Silvia Sörensen Rachel Missell、Alexander Eustice-Corwin和 **Dorine Otieno**在发表的文章中探讨了老龄化相关准备（**ARP**）的视角。文章聚焦于理解社会政策背景下老龄化相关准备（ARP）的前因和结果。他们区分了四个不同领域中的规划：退休、住房、未来护理需求、以及临终护理的预先指示。他们指出，甚至在老年人认为是总体计划的那些方面也几乎没有具体的规划。许多老年人不重视脆弱性和护理需求日渐增加的可能性。预先护理规划更为常见，因为其是医疗系统的指令。居住在社区的老年人对其未来需求的总体计划作了报告，但没有具体提到如何实现这些计划。仅有

1%-5%的老年人报告称拥有关于护理的具体计划（Black et al. 2008）。作者指出，尽管执行了预先指示，但对这些指示的理解却并不清晰。Boaz的住院经历就是这样的情况。老龄化相关准备的主要障碍包括不充足的内外部资源。结构性障碍包括禁止重要护理规划的现有政策。作者就提升目标设定提供建议，将目标设定作为有用的个体策略，并结合更年龄友好型的环境，后者为有效规划提供结构性支持。

在监狱中老去是作者**Tina Maschi、Keith Morgen、Annette Hintenach、Adriana Kaye**和 **Karen Bullock**的文章主题。他们深入概述了全球老龄化监狱人口和该群体的相关问题（例如身体虚弱、早期死亡、老年痴呆风险）。这篇文章提出一个从竞争和冲突模式到关爱的正义伙伴关系（CJP）模式的范式转变，前者聚焦于惩罚和报复，后者推崇一个更具人文关怀的响应方式。Maschi等人提出的CJP模式的目标是"在生命最具考验的时刻和经历中推动、促进、支持、庆祝对他人的关怀。"作者主张，这样的响应对那些老龄的、残疾的、正在监狱中死去的人而言更为人道，并且对例如那些遭遇无家可归、自然或人为灾害的其他社区具有相关性。尽管犯人和重症住院病人看似没有什么共同之处，但难以逃避的事实是，医院都存在完全遵循制度的共同性质，并且显示了集体的、分离的、以及制度性的管理特征（Goffman, 1958）。

Richard Johnson的文章有关于退休期间黑人-白人在财务安全方面的差距。他指出贫困人群收入保护中存在的不足，尤其是少数种族，他们在退休期间主要依赖社会保障金。年轻黑人更加受限的就业机会还导致了晚年生活的财务不安全。政策建议包括支持社会保障金和社会安全生活补助金（SSI）支付。作者还呼吁为年轻少数种族提供更好的机会，以实现住房自有并提升收入，以期在老年能更安稳。增加最低福利是值得的，因为这将帮助最困难的接受者。政府财政投资更小的额外措施包括"确保黑人在信用、住房和劳动市场受到公正的对待。"

《区分年龄**VS.**整合年龄：新自由主义政策和生命历程的未来》的作者是**Dale Dannefer、Jielu Lin**和**George Gonos**。文章聚焦于更加宏观-社会的现象。作者详细审视了区分年龄的制度化三段式生命历程和由学者Matilda Riley提出的整合年龄的替代方案。文章分析了新自由主义式社会政策（例如商业放松管制、公共服务的私有化、减税、以及社会福利计划的削减）对生命历程（教育、工作、退休）产生的破坏性影响。文章向读者描述了一系列政策变革，这些变革有可能以提升个体和群体福祉的方式重建制度性的生命历程。这些变革包括与下列相关的政策：普遍基本收入、小额债券提议、生活收入要求、累进税政策、以及免费的大学教育。作者所倡导的改革还对临终医疗的提升作出承诺。

将本期*JEP*收录的文章置于政策、实践和老年人生活经历的情境下

本期*JEP*收录的文章呼吁关注晚年生活需求的深度与广度。虽然这类需求要求政策和实践的进步，但也要求在现有政策执行过程中顾及"常见礼

仪"（common decency）这一简单概念（Schorr 1986）。缺少社会资本、金融资源和社会支持的那些人在应对生病带来的挑战和摸索医疗系统的时候面临特殊困难。种族歧视也将老年人置于特殊风险中（Williams, Neighbors & Jackson 2003）。

当个人脆弱性在临终前增加时，医疗系统和服务交付系统变得尤其具有挑战性。我希望，通过我在这篇社论中关于临终护理及丧失亲友之人的需求的个人反思，将鼓舞读者以经历上述政策倡议的老年人的有利视角，对本期收录的文章进行批判性评价。老年人不仅能从满足其个人需求和社会需求的政策中受益，他们的生活经历也需要与上述政策目标相匹配。鉴于政策和实践执行的不足，即便是最善意的政策也无法充分提升晚年生活质量。

在生命最虚弱的阶段，仅靠正式服务很有可能是不够的，并且老年人需要家人及密友的非正式支持。基于和这些人的强烈情感联系，脆弱的老年人能确信其自尊和需求将被满足。非正式支持网络的成员也更有可能熟悉脆弱老年人的价值观及偏好，并能努力满足甚至是表述不清的需求。结果则是，需要帮助的老年人及其家庭成员能作为正式服务和政策执行的有用指引。临终前尤为重要的是，从业人员与家庭成员及重要他人进行沟通，因为老年病人可能再也无法表达请求。

人文关怀是与在临终前提供悉心关怀（responsive care）最密切相关的概念。人文关怀被视为包括"一种由共情、情感支持和用于理解和减轻个体痛苦和顾虑的举措为特征的关系"（Mannion 2014, p.115）。Tehranineshat 等人（2019）的文献系统性回顾发现，人文关怀涉及员工的伦理观和精神观、有效交流、专业技能、以及与病人的积极接触。

医疗环境在使医生和护士能提供人文关怀方面发挥了重要作用（Christiansen et al. 2015）。为理解"帮助脆弱老年人的政策"与"服务接受者的生活经历"之间的联系，也很重要的是，对关键医疗提供者的视角、经历和自主权加以衡量（Friedberg et al. 2014）。如果内科医生、护士和其他医疗专业人士能在工作的同时保持专业自主权，病人的医疗经历则很有可能得以改善。员工教育计划已因推动人文关怀而被提及，但这些计划似乎没有医疗机构对人文关怀所赋予的价值重要。

正如我之前所提到的，我的已故丈夫Boaz曾是一名相信科学研究和敬业教育能改善世界，尤其是老年人生活的乐观主义者。我在这篇社论中的结论也同意这一乐观主义，并表达了希望，即《老年政策期刊》收录的文章能最终有助于提升老年人的生活经历。正如Boaz恰当提出的那样，"我们从每一次经历中学习并需要将我们所学充分用于帮助他人。"

References

Binstock, R. H. (1989) Introduction to Journal of Policy Studies. Case Western Reserve University.

Constand, M. K., MacDermid, J. C., Dal Bello-Haas, V., & Law, M. (2014). Scoping review of patient-centered care approaches in healthcare. *BMC Health Services Research, 14*(1), 271.

Crawford, P., Brown, B., Kvangarsnes, M., & Gilbert, P. (2014). The design of compassionate care. *Journal of Clinical Nursing, 23*(23-24), 3589-3599.

Friedberg, M. W., Chen, P. G., Van Busum, K. R., Aunon, F., Pham, C., Caloyeras, J., ... & Crosson, F. J. (2014). Factors affecting physician professional satisfaction and their implications for patient care, health systems, and health policy. *Rand health quarterly, 3*(4).

Gawande, A. (2014). *Being mortal: Medicine and what matters in the end.* Metropolitan Books.

Gerteis, M. (1993). Through the patient's eyes: understanding and promoting patient-centered care. Jossey – Bass, San Francisco.

Goffman, E. (1958). Characteristics of total institutions. In *Symposium on preventive and social psychiatry* (pp. 43-84). US Government Printing Office.

Henderson, A., Van Eps, M. A., Pearson, K., James, C., Henderson, P., & Osborne, Y. (2009). Maintainance of patients' dignity during hospitalization: Comparison of staff–patient observations and patient feedback through interviews. *International Journal of Nursing Practice, 15*(4), 227-230.

Jeffrey, D. (2016). Empathy, sympathy and compassion in healthcare: Is there a problem? Is there a difference? Does it matter? Journal of the Royal Society of Medicine, 109(12), 446-452.

Jennings, B., Ryndes, T., D'Onofrio, C. A. R. O. L., & Baily, M. A. (2010). Access to hospice care: Expanding boundaries, overcoming barriers. *Palliative care: Transforming the care of serious illness,* 159-164.

Kahana, B., Dan, A., Kahana, E., & Kercher, K. (2004). The personal and social context of planning for end-of-life care. *Journal of the American Geriatrics Society, 52*(7), 1163-1167.

Kahana, E., Kahana, B., Lovegreen L,. Kahana J., Brown, J. & Kulle D. (2011). Health-care consumerism and access to health care: educating elders to improve both preventive and end-of-life care. *Research in the Sociology of Health Care, 29,* 173-193.

Kahana, E., Kahana, B., & Wykle, M. (2010). "Care-getting": A conceptual model of marshalling support near the end of life. *Current Aging Science, 3*(1), 71-78.

Kahana, E., Stange, K., Meehan, R., & Raff, L. (1997). Forced disruption in continuity of primary care: the patients' perspective. *Sociological Focus, 30*(2), 177-187.

Kneafsey, R., Brown, S., Sein, K., Chamley, C., & Parsons, J. (2016). A qualitative study of key stakeholders' perspectives on compassion in healthcare and the development of a framework for compassionate interpersonal relations. *Journal of Clinical Nursing, 25*(1-2), 70-79.

Mannion, R. (2014). Enabling compassionate healthcare: perils, prospects and perspectives. *International Journal of Health Policy and Management, 2*(3), 115

Nolan, M. T., & Mock, V. (2004). A conceptual framework for end-of-life care: A reconsideration of factors influencing the integrity of the human person. *Journal of Professional Nursing, 20*(6), 351-360.

Salamon, J. (2008). *Hospital: man, woman, birth, death, infinity, plus red tape, bad behavior, money, God, and diversity on steroids.* Penguin.

Saultz, J. W., & Lochner, J. (2005). Interpersonal continuity of care and care outcomes: a critical review. *The Annals of Family Medicine, 3*(2), 159-166.

Schorr, A. L. (1986). *Common decency: Domestic policies after Reagan.* Yale University Press.

Singer, P. A., Martin, D. K., & Kelner, M. (1999). Quality end-of-life care: patients' perspectives. *JAMA, 281*(2), 163-168.

Sweet, V. (2013). *God's Hotel: A Doctor, a Hospital, and a Pilgrimage to the Heart of Medicine.* Penguin.

Tehranineshat, B., Rakhshan, M., Torabizadeh, C., & Fararouei, M. (2019). Compassionate care in healthcare systems: a systematic review. *Journal of the National Medical Association, 111*(5), 546-554.

Warren, M. G., Weitz, R., & Kulis, S. (1998). Physician satisfaction in a changing health care environment: the impact of challenges to professional autonomy, authority, and dominance. *Journal of Health and Social Behavior,* 356-367.

White, H. L., & Glazier, R. H. (2011). Do hospitalist physicians improve the quality of inpatient care delivery? A systematic review of process, efficiency and outcome measures. *BMC Medicine, 9*(1), 58.

Williams, D. R., Neighbors, H. W., & Jackson, J. S. (2003). Racial/ethnic discrimination and health: Findings from community studies. *American Journal of Public Health, 93*(2), 200-208.

Youngson, R. (2011). Compassion in healthcare—the missing dimension of healthcare reform. Caregiver stress and staff support in illness, dying, and bereavement, 49-61.

The Elder Abuse Policy Landscape in the United States

Georgia J. Anetzberger, PhD, ACSW, FGSA

Case Western Reserve University and Consultant in Private Practice

gja3@case.edu

ABSTRACT

Elder abuse has been seen as a complex problem of potentially severe consequence to its victims for more than a half century. Therefore, not surprisingly, it is believed that only a multidisciplinary response is appropriate. The background and perspective of no single discipline or system alone seems sufficient. In the decades that followed initial problem recognition, elder abuse policy evolved, taking on the philosophies and approaches of the various disciplines or systems that assumed key roles in addressing the issue, namely social work, Aging Network, family violence programming, justice, and health care and promotion. This article, along with identifying and describing representative elder abuse policies, presents each of these disciplines or systems. Later two sets of policy recommendations are cited—National Policy Summit on Elder Abuse and Elder Justice Roadmap—that have been instrumental in providing elder abuse policy direction since 2000. Finally, challenges and opportunities are listed for current and future policy efforts, followed by special notation on the necessity of securing adequate funding for effective policy implementation.

Keywords: Adult Protective Services, Older Americans Act, Elder Justice Act, Elder Justice Roadmap, National Policy Summit on Elder Abuse

El paisaje de la política de abuso de ancianos en Estados Unidos

RESUMEN

El abuso de ancianos se ha considerado un problema complejo de consecuencias potencialmente graves para sus víctimas durante más de medio siglo. Por lo tanto, no es sorprendente que se crea que solo una respuesta multidisciplinaria es apropiada. El trasfondo y

 doi: 10.18278/jep.1.2.2

la perspectiva de ninguna disciplina o sistema por sí solos parecen suficientes. En las décadas que siguieron al reconocimiento inicial del problema, la política de abuso de personas mayores evolucionó, asumiendo las filosofías y enfoques de las diversas disciplinas o sistemas que asumieron roles clave para abordar el problema, a saber, trabajo social, Red de Envejecimiento, programación de violencia familiar, justicia y salud. atención y promoción. Este artículo, junto con la identificación y descripción de las políticas representativas de abuso de ancianos, presenta cada una de estas disciplinas o sistemas. Posteriormente, se citan dos conjuntos de recomendaciones de políticas, la Cumbre Nacional de Políticas sobre Abuso de Ancianos y la Hoja de Ruta de Justicia de Ancianos, que han sido fundamentales para proporcionar una dirección de política de abuso de ancianos desde 2000. Por último, se enumeran los desafíos y oportunidades para los esfuerzos políticos actuales y futuros, seguidos de notación sobre la necesidad de asegurar el financiamiento adecuado para la implementación efectiva de políticas.

Palabras clave: Abuso de ancianos, Servicios de protección para adultos, Justicia de ancianos

关于虐待老年人的美国政策概况

摘要

大半个世纪以来，虐待老年人一直被视为一个对受害者造成潜在严重后果的复杂问题。因此，意料之中的是，只有多学科响应措施是适宜的。不仅仅依靠单个学科或系统的背景和视角似乎是足够的。自最初发现该问题的几十年后，与虐待老人相关的政策经历了演变，吸收了不同学科或系统的理念和方法，这些学科或系统在应对该问题时发挥了关键作用，即社会工作、老龄化网络（Aging Network）、家庭暴力防治计划（family violence programming）、正义、医疗及其推广。本文在识别和描述代表性老年人虐待政策的同时，还展现了这些学科及系统。随后引用了两套政策建议—关于虐待老年人的国家政策峰会（National Policy Summit on Elder Abuse）和老年人正义蓝图（Elder Justice Roadmap）—自2000年以来，它们在提供老年人虐待政策方向上发挥了重要作用。最后，列举了当前和未来政策举措的挑战和机遇，随后特别记录了为有效政策执行而确保充足资金的必要性。

关键词：虐待老年人，成年人保护服务，老年人正义

Introduction

> "Physical impairments and social losses make older people highly vulnerable to crime and abuse. While much has been written about the elderly's susceptibility to crime, the problem of abuse by relatives and caretakers in the community has been largely neglected .... [It] requires enough attention to initiate large scale action in legislation and effective programming."
>
> —From an article presenting findings from the first elder abuse research, initiated in 1977 by Elizabeth Lau and Jordan Kosberg, Cleveland, Ohio social workers (Lau & Kosberg, 1979, pp. 11, 15).

Elder abuse is complex and assumes many forms. Although proposed definitions of it lack universal acceptance and use, there is considerable agreement that minimally the problem involves intentional harm, suffering, or loss inflicted on an older adult by a trusted other, such as a family member or paid caregiver (National Research Council, 2003; Centers for Disease Control and Prevention, 2016; World Health Organization, 2020). Likewise, its forms generally are thought to include physical, emotional, financial, and sexual abuse, as well as neglect (Hall, Karch, & Crosby, 2016; Jackson 2018). Some experts, however, suggest a broader conceptualization of elder abuse that includes self-neglect and self-abuse, perhaps along with fraud and scams by acquaintances and strangers (Anetzberger, 2012; Dong, 2014). Others identify subsets of the problem. For example, those concerned with domestic violence in later life concentrate on domestic violence and sexual assault experienced by older adults (Crockett, Brandl, & Dabby, 2015; Administration for Community Living, 2020a).

Elder abuse also is widespread and occurs across settings. A large-scale nationally representative prevalence study suggests that one in ten community-dwelling older adults experienced elder abuse the previous year (Acierno, Hernandez, Amstadter, Resnick, Steve, Muzzy, & Kilpatrick, 2010). Elder abuse occurrence was highest for financial abuse (5.2%) and neglect (5.1%) and lowest for physical abuse (1.6%) and sexual abuse (<1.0%). The perpetrators usually were intimate partners, adult offspring, or other family members. In addition, elder abuse was more likely when victims had low social support, were dependent on others, had experienced prior trauma, or had poor health status. Other studies reveal that its prevalence may be greater (though yet unknown) for certain sub-populations, such as older adults with dementia or cognitive impairment (Wigglesworth, Mosqueda, Mulnard, Liao, Gibbs, & Fitzgerald, 2010; Dong, Chen, & Simon, 2014) and those residing in long-term care facilities (Rosen, Pillemer, & Lachs, 2008; Castle & Beach, 2013). Further, sizable numbers of elder abuse victims experience poly-victimization (i.e., more than one form simultaneously), for instance, 30-40% of those reported to adult protective services (APS) (Teaster et al., 2006; Clancy, McDaid, O'Neill, & O'Brien, 2011).

Finally, despite the serious effects it can have on victims, elder abuse is seldom reported to authorities charged to assist. New York state prevalence research found that only one in 24 elder abuse situations was reported, with rates particularly low for neglect (one in 57) and financial abuse (one in 44) (Lachs & Berman, 2011). The possible reasons for lack of reporting are many and varied. They include not knowing how to report or to whom, client confidentiality considerations, belief that the situation is a family matter, and lack of faith in those charged with abuse investigation (Schmeidel, Daly, Rosenbaum, Schmuch, & Jogerst, 2012; DeLiema, Navarro, Enguidanos, & Wilbur, 2015). Moreover, diverse populations, such as sexual and ethnic minorities, may prefer other sources of assistance, for example, friends or family members (Westwood, 2019; Li, Chen, & Dong, 2020). Lastly, research indicates the morbidity and mortality of elder abuse. Victims experience higher rates of health problems, depression and anxiety, and risk of death than non-victims (Podnieks & Thomas, 2017; Yunus, Hairi, & Choo, 2019).

From the above description of elder abuse, it should not be surprising that policy at all government levels has been seen as essential for problem identification, prevention, and treatment. The sections which follow discuss the evolution of elder abuse public policy in the United States both historically and currently from the various lenses it has assumed. Key federal and state laws are identified, and their major provisions described under the various problem perspectives which have framed elder abuse intervention. In addition, important advocates and organizations are named for each perspective. Then efforts aimed at recommending federal policy are considered along with their successes and shortcomings. The article ends with a summary of challenges and opportunities for elder abuse policy moving forward.

Policy Evolution

"Senator Pepper and Senator Pryor, I want to personally thank you for holding this hearing concerning the pervasive problem of elder abuse. This subject has been a major concern of mine for almost 2 years and our office has done considerable research to arrive at legislative solutions to this most serious national problem .... The 'Adult Abuse Prevention and Treatment Act' which we are introducing today, will create a National Center on Adult Abuse and will provide money to States for adult abuse prevention and treatment program. In order to qualify for these funds, States must have in effect an adult abuse, neglect, and exploitation law which provides for mandatory reporting and immunity for persons reporting ....

—Prepared statement of Ohio Representative Mary Rose Oakar during the first joint Congressional hearing devoted exclusively to elder abuse committed by family members (U.S. Senate Special Committee on Aging and U.S. House Select Committee on Aging, 1980, p. 12).

The development of elder abuse policy reflects changes in issue framing and discipline or system dominance over time. Collectively such policy aims to prevent elder abuse, protect the victim or at-risk older adult, and prosecute the perpetrator. It should not be surprising that many different disciplines or systems have assumed roles in elder abuse policy development. As evident in the preceding section, the problem's complexity, scope, and consequences demand a variety of professional backgrounds and skills for detection, assessment, and intervention (Anetzberger, 2005, 2011; O'Brien-Suric, Benson, Dong, & Fulmer, 2017). Indeed, the importance of a multidisciplinary approach to elder abuse was recognized from the earliest days of problem recognition and response (U.S. Department of Health, Education, and Welfare, 1961; Hall & Mathiasen, 1968). The popularity of this approach has exploded in recent times, evident in the growth of state and local elder abuse networks and multidisciplinary teams nationwide (U.S. Department of Justice, 2020). Although most professionals in the field of elder abuse applaud a multidisciplinary approach for its potential to improve communication and working relations, it has always carried the possibility to ignite suspicion, competition, and even division within networks, teams, and even the field itself. The approach has resulted in a steady growth of elder abuse policies at all government levels, reflecting varying philosophies and objectives, and unfortunately sometimes also creating confusion and disillusionment among those trying to understand and apply them to specific abuse situations.

Policy development began more than a half century ago. At the time elder abuse was usually seen as a social problem centered on self-neglect and potential exploitation, with social workers most vocal about taking action to stop it. Mid-twentieth century America witnessed increasing numbers of older adults. They often lived alone in urban centers without nearby family for help. Some had cognitive impairment. Community leaders, particularly those from social service agencies, believed that protective care was required to ensure their safety and well-being (Cole, 1962; Ross, 1968). Ultimately this resulted in passage of state APS statutes and supportive federal policy in the form of Title XX of the Social Security Act beginning in the early 1970s.

Somewhat later elder abuse became an aging issue, with those in the

Aging Network assuming key advocacy roles. Starting in the 1970s with a focus on elder abuse in nursing homes, leaders within the Administration on Aging (AoA), state units on aging, and area agencies on aging led efforts to amend the Older Americans Act (OAA) of 1965 to become a primary vehicle for elder abuse prevention and response. This early concern about the mistreatment of nursing home residents arose from a series of exposes, which in turn led to hearings on the subject in the U.S. Senate (Mendelson, 1974; Townsend, 1970).

A third perspective originated when elder abuse first received problem recognition, during the late 1970s. However, it failed to imprint policy until the mid-1980s. Seeing the problem as an aspect of family violence, this perspective is associated with those from domestic violence and sexual assault programming. The recognition that older adults could be domestic violence victims was bolstered by large-scale research findings on their existence (e.g., Straus & Gelles, 1988; Pillemer & Finkelhor, 1988) as well as a forum on middle and later life battered women convened by AARP (AARP Women's Initiative, 1992). Related policy initiatives tended to take the form of amending established law to include older adults as a targeted population, illustrated by the Family Violence Prevention and Services Act and Violence Against Women Act.

Since the late 1980s elder abuse most often has been regarded as a crime, with the justice system in the forefront

of public policy development at both federal and state levels. The timing of this perspective coincides with the "tough on crime" political platforms of the 1980s, when criminal justice shifted away from rehabilitation toward crime control. In the aftermath, most states accelerated their use of incarceration, even for less serious offences (National Research Council, 2014). Although criminal laws long existed which could respond to some incidents of elder abuse, more recently legislatures have enacted statutes which provide criminal penalty for elder abuse infliction specifically. Lately particular attention has been given to financial exploitation, both in terms of enhanced penalty and encouragement of greater reporting of incidents. The latter focus is seen in recent passage of the federal Senior Safe Act, which allows financial institutions along with investment advisers and brokers to report financial exploitation without being sued, providing they have trained employees on appropriate detection of the problem. Most notable among federal elder abuse laws is the Elder Justice Act, which has both justice origins and notable justice provisions. It also has been heralded as the most comprehensive elder abuse policy to date.

Medical professionals and public health officials represent the latest discipline or system to assume a leadership role in elder abuse policy formation. Elder abuse has been seen as a medical syndrome since the mid-1970s (Butler, 1975) and a public health concern since the mid-1980s (U.S. Office of the Surgeon General, 1986). However, until recently those involved in health care and promotion have focused more on practice and research than on policy with regard to elder abuse. This perspective changed during the past two decades (Irving & Hall, 2018). Largely spurred by a growing interest in prevention within the field of elder abuse, the public health framework increasingly has been applied to elder abuse policy and program development (Nerenberg, 2008, 2019). Consequently, policy-oriented activities on elder abuse have emerged from the Centers on Disease Control and Prevention as well as other health-related sources (Teaster, Hall, & Zanghami, 2018).

Problem Perspectives Reflected in Policy

"This report is the first comprehensive analysis of the subject we have chosen to call elder abuse .... [It] concludes that elder abuse is an extremely serious, widespread and until now, largely hidden problem in the United States ... [and] that there is immediate need for action at both the State and Federal level to prevent the problem from occurring in the future."

—Preface to the first Congressional report on elder abuse, written by Claude Pepper, Chair of the U.S. House Committee on Aging (1981, p. III).

Social Problem

The earliest elder abuse policy sought to establish APS as an intervention for functionally impaired adults at risk or victims of abuse, neglect, or exploitation. This approach began in the aftermath of 1950s with U.S. Department of Health, Education, and Welfare support for protective services unit demonstration projects. In 1962 Title XVI of the Social Security Act was enacted, providing matching grants for local public welfare agencies to develop and implement APS, with later amendments requiring APS inclusion in all state plans. However, few states complied (U.S. Senate Special Committee on Aging, 1977). During this decade, too, select federal agencies offered grants to create and evaluate APS models. Recipient organizations included Cleveland's Benjamin Rose Institute and San Diego's Protective Services Agency (Blenkner, Bloom, Nielsen, & Weber, 1974; Horowitz & Estes, 1971). Program evaluation findings were disappointing and disturbing (e.g., "intensive service of the sort supplied in the project with a heavy reliance on custodial care may actually accelerate decline" (Blenkner et al., 1974, p. 183), but failed to stem the spread of APS nationwide.

Adult protective services expansion was stimulated by the passage in 1974 of Title XX of the Social Security Act. The law mandated programming and provided funds to address the goal of preventing or remedying child and vulnerable adult abuse, neglect, or exploitation. Around the same time, states (beginning with Nebraska and North Carolina in 1973) proceeded to enact APS legislation, partly in anticipation of federal funding. The statutes varied in specific provisions without federal directive and only later available model legislation (U.S. Senate Special Committee on Aging, 1977). Still, there were, and continues to be, certain commonalities among state laws (Meagher, 1993). By the end of the 1980s all states had APS laws (with some states having multiple such laws), and Title XX was block granted. Block granting gave states discretion in fund allocation, but eliminated any required fund use for APS. Nonetheless, Social Services Block Grant (SSBG) goals still include prevention of neglect, abuse, and exploitation for adults (and children) unable to protect themselves. Although fewer states allocate SSBG funds for APS than under Title XX, APS still receives the largest proportion of total SSBG expenditures targeting vulnerable and older adults (Gottlich, 1994; SSBG Annual Report, 2018).

Social service leadership in early elder abuse policy also is evident in other ways. For example, completing the first studies on the problem, social workers, like Elizabeth Lau and Jordan Kosberg, then helped raise it to an issue of national concern through testimony at Congressional hearings. In addition, the American Public Welfare Association received the first grant to administer the newly formed National Center on Elder Abuse in the late 1980s, appointing Toshio Tatara as director. In that context, he helped inform pub-

lic policy through such efforts as conducting the first national elder abuse incidence study and examining cultural dimensions for understanding and responding to the problem.

Today APS is the only nationwide program dedicated solely to an elder abuse response. Its core functions involve receiving and investigating reports or referrals of abuse, neglect, or exploitation; determining client status and service need; providing or arranging and coordinating services to prevent or treat maltreatment; and seeking legal intervention, if indicated (Liu & Anetzberger, 2019). As reflected in state law, APS programs are typically state administered, usually operating within departments of social or human services or units on aging, and employing social workers more often than other professionals. All programs investigate abuse, neglect, or exploitation in community settings, and more than half investigate those in residential settings as well (Quinn & Benson, 2012). Although anyone can make a report, usually specific persons, like health care providers and law enforcement, are required to report, except in New York, which lacks mandatory reporting provisions. State APS laws vary in other ways as well. Examples include the particular allegation that triggers reporting, definitions of maltreatment forms, classification of abuse as criminal or civil, timelines for reporting as well as commencing and completing the report investigation, client eligibility requirements, and abuse remedies.

Recently the federal Administration for Community Living (ACL) provided a national "home" for APS, in the process seeking to promote more commonality among state programs through such voluntary measures as a uniform reporting system, consensus guidelines, and innovation grants. A major source for policy information and advocacy on APS is the National APS Association, with policy leadership from William Benson.

Aging Issue

On the heels of the first White House Conference on Aging, the 1965 OAA was passed. It did so without means-tested provisions. The OAA is widely considered the premier federal policy for organizing and delivering social and nutrition services to older adults and their caregivers. It essentially creates a structure at federal, state, and local levels to plan, administer, and authorize grants for programming designed to foster the well-being and independence of older adults in their homes and communities. The OAA requires regular reauthorization and therefore provides periodic updating opportunity.

Early recognition of elder abuse as an issue of concern can be seen in OAA Title I Declaration of Objectives for Older Americans, which argues for protection against abuse, neglect, and exploitation. At various times in OAA history new provisions have stimulated significant activity toward the realization of this objective. Among the most notable amendments are the following: (1) 1978 requirement of each state to establish a long-term care ombudsman program to cover nursing homes (later

expanded to include other long-term care residences and settings, beginning in 1980 with board and care homes); (2) 1984 requirement of area agencies on aging to assess local need for elder abuse prevention services; (3) 1987 authorization of appropriations for the prevention of elder abuse, neglect, and exploitation along with provision to ombudsmen of direct and immediate access to residents for necessary protection and advocacy; and (4) 1992 creation of a new Title VII Vulnerable Elder Rights Activities, resulting in the consolidation and enhancement of programs like the long-term care ombudsman, elder abuse prevention, and legal assistance development, and elevating the role of local ombudsman programs as advocates for system change.

Other OAA titles further provide the means for addressing elder abuse. For example, Title III offers grant funding for services which could have the effect of reducing abuse risk factors, such as senior centers, congregate meals, and adult day care to curve social isolation. In addition, Title IV enables grant funding for research, demonstration, and other projects to promote better elder abuse response, among other aims. Illustration of such use is found in two of the earliest studies on elder abuse in private homes, undertaken during Fiscal Years 1978-1979 by the Universities of Michigan and Maryland (Cronin & Allen, 1982). Moreover, the first federal legislation on elder abuse (i.e., Prevention, Identification, and Treatment of Adult Abuse Act of 1981), discussed in the quotation that began this section and introduced in 1980 by Representatives

Mary Rose Oakar and Claude Pepper, included provision for what later would become the National Center on Elder Abuse (NCEA), through subsequent legislation in 1988. The NCEA received permanent home with AoA following 1992 amendments to the OAA (Teaster, Wangmo, & Anetzberger, 2010). It currently is the major national resource for information and training across elder abuse research, policy, and practice. For the last several years it has been directed by geriatrician Laura Mosqueda from the University of Southern California, in partnership with a wide range of organizations and diverse Advisory Board. In 2011 the National APS Resource Center also was created using discretionary grant funding.

In addition to OAA establishment and expansion of long-term care ombudsman programming, all states have passed laws supporting it, and some states also have enacted separate statutes aimed at resident abuse. Another important federal law with this purpose is the Omnibus Budget Reconciliation Act (OBRA) of 1987, which mandates nursing homes to preserve resident quality of life, defines resident abuse, fosters abuse prevention through health care worker education, and requires states to investigate resident abuse allegations. OBRA also mandates nursing homes to promote and protect resident rights, including the right to be free from physical or mental abuse, corporal punishment, involuntary seclusion, and physical or chemical restraint used for discipline or convenience. Finally, it requires that residents have direct and immediate access to an om-

budsman when protection and advocacy services are needed.

Interest in and activity directed at elder abuse within the Aging Network accelerated during the Obama Administration due to the seven-year leadership of Kathy Greenlee as Assistant Secretary of Aging and ACL Administrator. Among her accomplishments were those connected to providing a "home" for APS, as above described. In addition, she led agency efforts to publish final federal regulations for the long-term care ombudsman program and gave frequent national voice to the realities and scope of elder abuse. Her replacement under the Trump Administration, Lance Robertson, continued the priority given to the issue, considering protecting rights and preventing abuse among the five pillars he envisioned for the Aging Network (Administration for Community Living, 2020b). A major source for policy information and advocacy on elder abuse from an Aging Network perspective is the National Association of Area Agencies on Aging.

Aspect of Family Violence

The physical abuse of older Americans may have been "discovered" and described in scholarly publications by physicians somewhat earlier. However, the issue did not emerge as a matter worthy of federal government concern until a 1978 hearing on domestic violence convened by the U.S. House Select Committee on Aging and U.S. House Science and Technology Subcommittee. After testifying on the broad topic,

Suzanne Steinmetz, a noted family violence researcher from the University of Delaware, was asked whether or not she saw the abuse of older adults as a significant problem. She responded affirmatively, gave examples, and then predicted that "the 80s will be the decade of the battered parent" (Cravedi, 1986, p. 4). She was correct. Awareness and action on elder abuse dramatically increased during the 1980s, albeit largely outside of the family violence policy arena. During that decade the policy surge focused on battered young and middle-aged women, including the enactment in 1984 of both the Victims of Crime Act and Family Violence Prevention and Services Act and, a decade later, the Violence Against Women Act. Subsequent reauthorizations of each policy expanded their scope, including consideration of the needs of older women, often through recognition of them as an underserved population.

The three policies have interlocking general purposes. The Victims of Crime Act (VOCA) was established to provide funds for assisting and compensating survivors of crime of all ages. Funds are distributed as formula grants to states and territories for victim resources. Resources can include domestic violence shelters and other services, like counseling and emergency transportation, as well as compensation to victims for crime-related losses, such as medical costs and the replacement or repair of eyeglasses. Discretionary funds are used for national scope training and assistance, such as developing training curricula and conducting training of professionals who work in victim ser-

vices or allied fields. In addition to this federal policy, all states have adopted a victim bill of rights. The Family Violence Prevention and Services Act is the only federal funding source exclusively dedicated to domestic violence shelters and programs. It provides the most federal funding for domestic violence direct service providers. Among the programs that receive support locally are those that offer legal assistance, counseling, coalition building, and violence prevention education. Like VOCA, the Family Violence Prevention and Services Act distributes funds to states and territories that then make grants available to service providers. Furthermore, it funded the first National Elder Abuse Incidence Study in 1992. Finally, the Violence Against Women Act (VAWA) represents the first federal law that acknowledged domestic violence as a crime and provided federal funds to communities in order to encourage coordinated responses to address the problem. It also provides grants to help law enforcement combat violence against women, strengthens penalties, and prohibits activities that previously had not been recognized as illegal. In so doing, VAWA attempts to give states and communities the tools (e.g., training, services) that they need to respond effectively to domestic violence, sexual assault, and stalking, including that affecting women age 50 and older. In 2013, VAWA was amended to include the Victims of Trafficking and Violence Protection Act (originally passed in 2000), which enables the provision of assistance to, among others, older adult victims of involuntary servitude or slavery.

Besides federal law, all states have domestic violence laws that may apply to certain situations of elder abuse. The intent of such law is to provide legal recourse for victims experiencing domestic violence. States vary in their statute provisions, including the breath of definition given the problem and its forms, standards associated with the perpetrator's conduct, qualifying relationship between victim and perpetrator, and code placement. In general, domestic violence law contains criminal provisions aimed at punishing perpetrators and civil provisions offering protective orders for harmed victims. The National Clearinghouse on Abuse in Later Life is a major source for policy information and advocacy on elder abuse as an aspect of family violence, founded by Bonnie Brandl.

Crime

As mentioned earlier, general state criminal codes may apply to particular elder abuse situations, including those for battery, theft, and fraud. In some states, when the victim is an older adult, the penalties are increased. Additionally, beginning in the mid-1980s some states specified elder abuse as one or more distinct crimes.

At the federal level, two statutes are noteworthy for addressing elder abuse as primarily a justice matter. They are discussed in the remaining paragraphs of this section. Beyond these are still other statutes, perhaps less directly concerned with elder abuse, but potentially important for protecting select victims and prosecuting their perpetrators.

For example, under the Civil Rights of Institutionalized Persons Act, the U.S. Department of Justice can pursue civil rights cases against public long-term care facilities when providers abuse or neglect persons in their care or fail to meet residents' constitutional rights.

The Elder Justice Act (EJA) was introduced in 2002, and then went through multiple versions and Congressional considerations. It finally was enacted as an amendment to the Patient Protection and Affordable Care Act, signed into law in 2010. The EJA brought the term "elder justice" to the policy vernacular around elder abuse. Its aim is to establish a comprehensive and coordinated federal response to elder abuse that considers social service and public health approaches along with those of civil and criminal justice. EJA's key provisions were crafted by U.S. Senate Special Committee on Aging staff Lauren Fuller and Marie-Therese Connolly. Its eventual passage was significantly aided by the Elder Justice Coalition, an advocacy group led by Robert Blancato. Among those provisions are the following: authorization of $777 million over four years; enhancement of national elder justice coordination through establishment of an Elder Justice Coordinating Council and Advisory Board on Elder Abuse, Neglect, and Exploitation; strengthening of state APS operations through direct funding and training demonstration programs; provision of grants to forensic centers to develop elder abuse forensic markers and expertise; and requiring the U.S. Department of Health and Human Services to promulgate guidelines on human subject protection issues in elder abuse research. However, the primary emphasis of the EJA is on elder abuse in long-term care settings. Related provisions include: direct funding for long-term care ombudsman services and training as well as grants to improve facility staffing, the establishment of a National Training Institute for Surveyors, enhancing state survey agency investigation systems, supporting a study on establishing a national nurse aide registry, and funding background check programs targeting facility employees. Lastly, the EJA is regarded as the first federal law to state specifically that it is the right of older adults to be free of elder abuse.

The second federal elder justice policy of note was passed in 2017. Titled the Elder Abuse Prevention and Prosecution Act, its intent is to direct DOJ in ways that better prevent crimes against older adults, improve the treatment of elderly victims, investigate and prosecute elder abuse crimes, and enforce elder abuse laws. Toward these goals, the Act requires each federal judicial district to designate an elder justice coordinator, whose primary focus is on prosecuting elder abuse cases. It compels the implementation of comprehensive related training of Federal Bureau of Investigation agents. The Act authorizes: appointment of elder justice coordinators in DOJ and the Bureau of Consumer Protection, formation of a working group under the Attorney General's Advisory Committee to provide guidance on DOJ elder abuse policies and strategies, and grants for qualified state courts to evaluate adult

guardianship and conservatorship proceedings. Finally, it seeks to improve DOJ data collection and reporting on crimes against older adults as well as to provide training and technical assistance to state and local governments with the goal of improving their ability to investigate, prosecute, and prevent crimes against this population. The Elder Justice Initiative of DOJ is an important source of information on elder abuse as a justice issue and crime.

Health Concern

Public policy may not have been a dominant focus of health professionals interested in elder abuse until recently, but that does not mean elder abuse policy escaped their concern. A federal example is the Medicare and Medicaid Patient and Program Protection Act of 1987. The Act requires the Secretary of the U.S. Department of Health and Human Services to exclude from participation in Medicare, Medicaid, and SSBG any person or entity convicted of program-related abuse or neglect, with the exclusion mandatory and not able to be waived. Legislation passed a decade earlier established Medicaid Fraud Control Units, with state and local law enforcement authorized to investigate and prosecute cases of patient abuse in residential care facilities receiving federal health care funds. Moreover, some state licensure laws for health care providers delineate patient rights, including freedom from abuse or neglect. Beyond legislative action, the Centers for Disease Prevention and Control funded research in the 1990s that systematically assessed how elder abuse investigations were influenced by the content and characteristics of state statutes. More recently, the agency has provided uniform definitions and data elements for collecting elder abuse data within a public health surveillance framework. Finally, the Centers for Medicare and Medicaid Services incorporated a measurement of elder abuse within the Physician Quality Reporting System. The National Consumer Voice for Quality Long-Term Care is an effective policy advocate for elder abuse victims receiving long-term services in any setting.

Policy Recommendations

"Elder justice is a long unrecognized human and civil rights issue. It raises fundamental questions about how we value life and view suffering in old age. It is low-hanging policy fruit long gone unplucked where good policy is cheaper than bad .... And it's an issue where real federal leadership and a modest investment of resources—by Congress, the administration, and private funders—could have a profound impact, mitigating the suffering of millions of people and saving billions of dollars. But to date, despite these great and growing moral, demographic, and economic imperatives, we have seen scarce federal leadership or investment by any entity."

—Introduction to "High-Cost Blind Spot" by Marie-Therese Connolly, JD, Senior Scholar at the Woodrow Wilson International Center for Scholars and architect of the Elder Justice Act (Connolly, 2012, p. 8).

There is a long history of making recommendations on elder abuse policy issues and needs. Most early efforts were offered by individuals in the form of either published article or legislative testimony. John Poertner (1987, pp. 412, 416, 420) exemplifies the former in his chapter on state policy options, in which he recommends: "careful problem definition [for] sound public policy development [...] creative solutions ... that protect victims in their environment or in the least restrictive environment," and "[use of] a narrow target population covering physical abuse and intentional neglect." Rosalie Wolf's (1989) testimony before Congress on the federal response to elder abuse illustrates the latter. In it, she makes nine recommendations, most toward enhancing existing law, such as the Family Violence Prevention and Services Act and SSBG, or providing funding for existing programs, like APS and in-home preventive services. Additionally, she proposes a national data reporting system, proclamation of an annual elder abuse prevention week, and use of the next White House Conference on Aging to mobilize a nationwide prevention program.

The National Policy Summit on Elder Abuse was held in 2001, a decade after these early proposals and a first-ever such event. It also later triggered similar local efforts in select states, such as New York and Ohio (Anetzberger, Breckman, Caccamise, Freeman, & Nerenberg, 2020). Convened by the NCEA and attended by approximately eighty experts, the Summit was charged with recommending a national policy agenda for protecting vulnerable older adults. Working groups across seven topics identified 21 consensus recommendations, which were then subjected to a process that resulted in ten priority items for the final action agenda. Identified priority items are listed in Figure 1. Assessing progress made on these recommendations since 2001 suggests that the majority have been realized, although perhaps not entirely as envisioned. More specifically, NCEA and its partners provide ongoing communications on elder abuse, the EJA was enacted, DOJ's Elder Justice Initiative alone is testament of the considerable progress made within the justice system, elder abuse education and training curricula are available from multiple sources from professional associations to universities, a national APS resource center exists, and the Elder Justice Coordinating Council fosters coordination among federal agencies with an elder abuse responsibility. Less evidence of accomplishment surrounds the expansion of age-appropriate mental health services and a National Institute on Aging commitment to elder abuse research. On the other hand, the National Institute of Justice has helped a

good deal in supporting such studies. In addition, there have been no Executive Order on policy review toward better coordination among responsible agencies and no Governmental Accountability Office study of the relationship between federal expenditures and elder abuse service needs.

Since 2001, several instances have occurred when elder abuse experts convened and developed policy recommendations. Most were small scale responses to looming policy opportunities, such as the 2015 White House Conference on Aging (Kaplan & Pillemer, 2015) and election of a new President (Mostada, Hirst, & Sabatino, 2016-17). However, the largest scale effort to date occurred in 2014, received funding from DOJ, and resulted in the Elder Justice Roadmap (EJR). An ambitious endeavor, the project solicited the perspectives of 750 stakeholders for concept mapping critical priorities in research, education, direct services, and, of course, policy; facilitated discussions with experts on related topics, like caregiving and diminished capacity; conducted leadership interviews with public officials and thought leaders on gaining traction for implementing an elder justice agenda; and compiled a project bibliography and resource listing relevant to the 122 identified priorities. Figure 1 presents the EJR first wave policy action items and policy priorities. Evaluating impact is more difficult for the EJR than for the National Policy Summit on Elder Abuse. In comparison to the Summit, the EJR's action items tend to be numerous rather than limited, sweeping instead of specified, and aspiration more than measurable. That said, unlike the Summit the EJR concluded with formation of a Steering Committee to disseminate the project document and encourage implementation of its priorities. The Committee met for over five years, tracking deliverables resulting from the EJR. For policy these include an elder justice focus at the 2015 White House Conference on Aging, a monograph on planning elder abuse multidisciplinary teams, and establishment of more than one hundred new elder abuse networks.

Policy Challenges and Opportunities

"The attempt to force the multiplicity of difficult human situations faced by older persons into an elder abuse framework is a waste of valuable time and energy that makes no sense for intervention, is not feasible politically, and could increase the risks faced by certain older persons. Instead, our attention should be directed to maintaining and expanding income protection measures, medical care provisions, and social service programs already in place at the federal and state levels."

—A "Guest Editor's Perspective" from James Callahan, Jr., Director of the Policy Center on Aging at Brandeis University, for a special journal issue on elder abuse (Callahan, 1986, p. 3).

Despite decades of legislative action across multiple domains, elder abuse policy still lags behind other areas of family violence and many aging-related concerns, like Alzheimer's disease and family caregiving. The most heralded deficit is funding, notably the lack of any dedicated federal revenue stream for APS and the minimal amount actually appropriated for EJA implementation, less than $60 million since policy enactment, although $777 million over four years was authorized. The Government Accountability Office (2011) calculated that federal agency spending on elder abuse in 2009 totaled $11.9 million in contrast to $649 million for violence against women programs. Little has changed in the funding contrast between elder abuse and other aspects of family violence since publication of the report. Furthermore, certain policies routinely appear "threatened with extinction," especially the SSBG (regularly faced with fund elimination) and the EJA (since 2014 up for reauthorization, and still waiting at the time of writing this article, more than a half decade later). Nonetheless, funding for elder abuse policy has improved somewhat over time, particularly in the following areas: DOJ initiatives, programs which fall under the domestic violence umbrella, and ACL APS/elder justice activities. Figure 2 lists various challenges to the elevation of elder abuse policy, fulfillment of related advocacy agendas, and obtainment of sufficient funding for program implementation.

The quotation beginning this section provides a stepping-off point for identifying opportunities to promote and improve elder abuse policy. In a sense, James Callahan urges advocates to move from a narrow focus on elder abuse to broader elder justice concerns in order to ensure that the needs of older adults are met and risk factors for elder abuse are diminished. This message is contained in recent communication recommendations on elder abuse from the FrameWorks Institute (2020), contracted by NCEA to improve understanding about the problem and so create a climate where it can be better addressed. The danger of reframing elder abuse in this manner lies in loss of focus on the problem altogether. After all, elder justice incorporates a wide range of individual rights, not simply freedom from elder abuse. Fortunately, opportunity for elder abuse policy enhancement exists in other ways, including those listed in Figure 3. Still, policy making is always a journey, with potential challenges and opportunities at every juncture. In the area of elder abuse, it is likely a journey without end, since eradicating the problem is more wishful thinking than probable reality. It is also a journey worth taking, if not for ethical considerations, then for the very meaning of society.

References

AARP Women's Initiative. (1993). *Abused elders or older battered women? Report on the AARP forum, October 29-30, 1992.* Washington, DC: AARP.

Acierno, R., Hernandez, M.A., Amstadter, A.B., Resnick, H.S., Steve. K., Muzzy, W., & Kilpatrick, D.G. (2010). Prevalence and correlates of emotional, physical, sexual, and financial abuse and potential neglect in the United States: The National Elder Mistreatment Study. *American Journal of Public Health,* 100(2), 292-297. https://doi.org/10.2105/ajph.2009.163089

Administration for Community Living (2020a). Late life domestic violence. Retrieved from https://acl.gov/programs/protections-rights-and-preventing-abuse/elder-justice/late-life-domestic-violence

Administration for Community Living. (2020b). *Administrator's pillars.* Retrieved from https://acl.gov/about-acl/administrators-pillars

Anetzberger, G.J. (2012). An update on the nature and scope of elder abuse. *Generations,* 36(3), 12-20. https://doi.org/10.4324/9780203049495

Anetzberger, G.J. (2011). The evolution of a multidisciplinary response to elder abuse. *Marquette Elder's Advisor,* 13(1), 107-128.

Anetzberger, G.J. (Ed.). (2005). *The clinical management of elder abuse.* Binghamton, NY: The Haworth Press. https://doi.org/10.1300/j018v28n01_02

Anetzberger, G.J., Breckman, R., Caccamise, P.L., Freeman, I.C., & Nerenberg, L. (2020). Building a national elder justice movement state by state: The promise of a national network of state elder justice coalitions. *Generations*, 44(1), 111-116. https://doi.org/10.1891/9780826147578

Blenkner, M., Bloom, M., Nielsen, M., & Weber, R. (1974). *Final report: Protective services for older people.* Cleveland, OH: The Benjamin Rose Institute. https://doi.org/10.1093/sw/21.2.162

Butler, R.N. (1975). *Why survive? Being old in America.* New York: Harper & Row. https://doi.org/10.1093/sw/21.4.341-c

Callahan, J.J. Jr. (1986). Guest editor's perspective. *Pride Institute Journal of Long Term Home Health Care*, 5(4), 2-3.

Castle, N., & Beach, S. (2013). Elder abuse in assisted living. *Journal of Applied Gerontology*, 32(2), 248-267. https://doi.org/10.1177/0733464811418094

Centers for Disease Control and Prevention. (2016). *Elder abuse surveillance: Uniform definitions and recommended core data elements.* Atlanta, GA: National Center for Injury Prevention and Control, Division of Violence Prevention.

Clancy, M., McDaid, B., O'Neill, D. & O'Brien, J.G. (2011). National profiling of elder abuse referrals. *Age and Ageing*, 40, 346-352. https://doi.org/10.1093/ageing/afr023

Cole, H.B. (1962, October 22). *Older persons in need of protective services.* Unpublished manuscript.

Connolly, M-T. (2012). High-cost blind spot. *Public Policy & Aging Report*, 22(1), 8-16. https://doi.org/10.1093/ppar/22.1.8

Connolly, M-T., Brandl, B., & Breckman, R. (2014). *The Elder Justice Roadmap: A stakeholder initiative to respond to an emerging health, justice, financial and social crisis.* Washington, D.C.: U.S. Department of Justice.

Cravedi, K.G. (1986). Elder abuse: The evaluation of federal and state policy reform. *Pride Institute Journal of Long Term Home Health Care*, 5(4), 4-9.

Crockett, C., Brandl, B., & Dabby, F.C. (2015). Survivors in the margins: The invisibility of violence against older women. *Journal of Elder Abuse & Neglect*, 27, 291-302. https://doi.org/10.1080/08946566.2015.1090361

Cronin, R., & Allen, B. (1982, April). *The uses of research sponsored by the Administration on Aging (AoA), Case study no. 5: Maltreatment and abuse of the elderly.* Washington, D.C.: American Gerontological Research Institute.

DeLiema, M., Navarro, A., Enguidanos, S., & Wilber, K. (2015). Voices from the frontlines: Examining elder abuse from multiple professional perspectives. *Health & Social Work, 40,* e15-e24. https://doi.org/10.1093/hsw/hlv012

Dong, X. (2014). Elder abuse: Research, practice, and health policy. The 2012 GSA Maxwell Pollack Award lecture. *The Gerontologist, 54*(2), 153-162. https://doi.org/10.1093/geront/gnt139

Dong, X., Chen, R., & Simon, M.A. (2014). Elder abuse and dementia: A review of the research and health policy. *Health Affairs, 33*(4), 642-649. https://doi.org/10.1377/hlthaff.2013.1261

FrameWorks Institute. (2020). *Talking elder abuse: A FrameWorks communications toolkit.* Retrieved from https://www.frameworksinstitute.org/toolkits/el derabuse/elements/items/elder-abuse-bp-quick-start-guide.pdf

Gottlich, V. (1994). Beyond granny bashing: Elder abuse in the 1990s. *Clearinghouse Review, 28*(4), 371-387.

Hall, G., & Mathiasen, G. (Ed.). (1968). *Overcoming barriers to protective services for the aged: Conference proceedings.* New York, NY: National Council on the Aging.

Hall, J., Karch, D.L., & Crosby, A. (2016). *Elder abuse surveillance: Uniform definitions and recommended core data elements.* Atlanta, GA: Centers for Disease Control and Prevention.

Horowitz, G., & Estes, C. (1971, May). *Protective services for the aged.* Washington, D.C.: U.S. Department of Health, Education, and Welfare.

Irving, S.M., & Hall, J.E. (2018). Elder abuse and the core function of public health: Using the 10 essential public health services as a framework for addressing elder abuse. In P.B. Teaster & J.E. Hall (Eds.), *Elder abuse and the public's health* (pp. 19-44). New York, NY: Springer Publishing Company. https://doi.org/10.1891/9780826171351.0002

Jackson, S.L. (2018). *Understanding elder abuse: A clinician's guide.* Washington, D.C.: American Psychological Association. https://doi.org/10.1037/0000056-000

Kaplan, D.B., & Pillemer, K. (2015). Fulfilling the promise of the Elder Justice Act: Priority goals for the White House Conference on Aging. *Public Policy & Aging Report, 25,* 63-66. https://doi.org/10.1093/ppar/prv001

Lachs, M.S., & Berman, J. (2011). *Under the radar: New York state elder abuse prevalence study.* New York, NY: William B. Hoyt Memorial New York State Children and Family Trust Fund, New York State Office of Children and Family Services.

Lau, E.E., & Kosberg, J.I. (1979, October). Abuse of the elderly by informal care providers. *Aging,* pp. 10-15.

Li, M., Chen, R., & Dong, X. (2020). Elder mistreatment across diverse cultures. *Generations,* 44(1), 20-25.

Lui, P-J, & Anetzberger, G.J. (2019). Adult protective services. In D. Gu & M.E. Dupre (Eds.), *Encyclopedia of gerontology and population aging.* Springer Nature Switzerland. http://doi.org/10.1007/978-3-319-69892-2_282-1

Meagher, M.S. (1993). Legal and legislative dimensions. In B. Byers & J.E. Hendricks (Eds.), *Adult protective services: Research and practice* (pp. 87-107). Springfield, IL: Charles C Thomas Publisher.

Mendelson, M.A. (1974). *Tender loving greed: How the incredibly lucrative nursing home "industry" is exploiting America's old people and defrauding us all.* New York, NY: Alfred A. Knopf.

Mills, W.L., Roush, R.E., Moye, J., Kunik, M.E., Wilson, N.L., Taffet, G.E., & Naik, A.D. (2012). An educational program to assist clinicians in identifying elder investment fraud and financial exploitation. *Gerontology & Geriatrics Education,* 33, 351-363. https://doi.org/10.1080/02701960.2012.702164

Mosqueda, L., Hirst, S., & Sabatino, C.P. (2016-2017). Strengthening elder safety and security. *Generations,* 40(4), 79-85.

Mulford, C.F., & Mao, A. (2017). Department of Justice: Elder maltreatment initiatives. In X. Dong (Ed.), *Elder abuse: Research, practice and policy* (pp. 637-651). Cham, Switzerland: Springer Nature.

National Center on Elder Abuse. (2002). *Proceedings: National Policy Summit on Elder Abuse.* Washington, D.C.: National Association of State Units on Aging.

National Research Council. (2014). *The growth of incarceration in the U.S.: Exploring causes and consequences.* Washington, D.C.: The National Academies Press. https://doi.org/10.17226/18613

National Research Council. (2003). *Elder mistreatment: Abuse, neglect, and exploitation in an aging America.* Panel to Review Risk and Prevalence of Elder Abuse and Neglect. R.J. Bonnie & R.B. Wallace, Eds. Washington, D.C.: The National Academies Press. https://doi.org/10.17226/10406

Nerenberg, L. (2019). *Elder justice, ageism, and elder abuse.* New York, NY: Springer Publishing Company. https://doi.org/10.1891/9780826147578

Nerenberg, L. (2008). *Elder abuse prevention: Emerging trends, and promising practices.* New York, NY: Springer Publishing Company. https://doi.

org/10.5860/choice.46-1199

O'Brien-Suric, N., Benson, A., Dong, X., & Fulmer, T. (2017). A multidisciplinary approach to the clinical management of elder abuse. In X. Dong (Ed.), *Elder abuse: Research, practice and policy* (pp. 215-228). Cham, Switzerland: Springer Nature. https://doi.org/10.1007/978-3-319-47504-2_11

Pillemer, K., & Finkelhor, D. (1988). The prevalence of elder abuse: A random sample survey. *The Gerontologist,* 28(1), 51-57. https://doi.org/10.1093/geront/28.1.51

Podneiks, E., & Thomas, C. (2017). The consequences of elder abuse. In X. Dong (Ed.), *Elder abuse: Research, practice and policy* (pp.109-123). Cham, Switzerland: Springer Nature. https://doi.org/10.1007/978-3-319-47504-2_6

Poertner, J. (1987). Elder abuse and neglect: Options for policy and practice. In G. Lesnoff-Caravaglia (Ed.), *Handbook of applied gerontology* (pp. 411-421). New York: Human Sciences Press.

Quinn, K.M., & Benson, W.F. (2012). The states' elder abuse victim services: A system still in search of support. *Generations,* 36(3), 66-72.

Rosen, T., Pillemer, K., & Lachs, M. (2008). Resident-to-resident aggression in long-term care facilities: An understudied problem. *Aggression and Violent Behavior,* 13(2), 77-87. https://doi.org/10.1016/j.avb.2007.12.001

Ross, H.A. (1968). Protective services for the aged. *The Gerontologist,* 8, 50-51. https://doi.org/10.1093/geront/8.1_part_2.50

Schmeidel, A.N., Daly, J.M., Rosenbaum, M.E., Schmuch, G.A., & Jogerst, G.J. (2012). Health care professionals' perspectives on barriers to elder abuse detection and reporting in primary care settings. *Journal of Elder Abuse & Neglect,* 24, 17-36. https://doi.org/10.1080/08946566.2011.608044

Stetson University. (2020). *Guide on adult protective services statutes.* Retrieved from http://www.stetson.edu/law/academics/elder/home/adult-protection-statues.php

Straus, M.A., & Gelles, R.J. (1988). How violent are American families? Estimates from the National Family Violence Resurvey and other studies. In G.T. Hotaling (Ed.), *Family violence and its consequences* (pp. 14-36). Newbury Park, CA: Sage Publications. https://doi.org/10.4324/9781315126401-8

Teaster, P.B., Hall, J.E., & Zarghami, F. (2018). Initiatives, organizations, and efforts addressing elder abuse. In P.B. Teaster & J. E. Hall (Eds.). *Elder abuse and the public's health* (pp. 153-180). New York, NY: Springer Publishing Company. https://doi.org/10.1891/9780826171351.0007

Teaster, P.B., Wangmo, T., & Anetzberger, G.J. (2010). A glass half full: The dubious history of elder abuse policy. *Journal of Elder Abuse & Neglect,* 22(1-2), 6-15. https://doi.org/10.1080/08946560903436130

Teaster, P.B., Dugar, T., Mendiondo, M., Abner, E., Cecil, K., & Otto, J. (2006). *The 2004 survey of state adult protective services: Abuse of adults 60 years of age and older.* Washington, D.C.: National Center on Elder Abuse.

Townsend, C. (1970). *Old age: The last segregation.* New York, NY: Grossman Publishers.

U.S. Department of Health, Education, and Welfare (1961). *The nation and its older people: Report of the White House Conference on Aging.* Washington, D.C.: U.S. Government Printing Office.

U.S. Department of Health and Human Services. (2020). SSBG final report FY2017. Retrieved at https://www.acf.hhs.gov/ocs/resource/ssbg-annual-report-fy-2017.

U.S. Department of Justice. (2020). *Elder justice networks locator map.* Retrieved at https://www.justice.gov/elderjustice/elder-justice-network-locator-map

U.S. Government Accountability Office. (2011). *Stronger federal leadership could enhance the response to elder abuse* (GAO-11-208) Washington, D.C.: Government Accountability Office.

U.S. House Select Committee on Aging (1981, April 18). *Elder abuse (An examination of a hidden problem).* Washington, D.C.: U.S. Government Printing Office.

U.S. Office of the Surgeon General. (1986). *Report: Surgeon General's workshop on violence and public health.* Washington, D.C.: U.S. Health Resources and Services Administration. https://doi.org/10.1037/e548712010-001

U.S. Senate Special Committee on Aging. (1977, July). *Protective services for the elderly: A working paper.* Washington, D.C.: U.S. Government Printing Office.

U.S. Senate Special Committee on Aging and U.S. House Select Committee on Aging. (1980, June 11). *Elder abuse.* Washington, D.C.: U.S. Government Printing Office.

Westwood, S. (2019). Abuse and older lesbian, gay, bisexual, and trans (LGBT) people: A commentary and research agenda. *Journal of Elder Abuse & Neglect,* 31, 97-114. https://doi.org/10.1080/08946566.2018.1543624

Wiglesworth, A., Mosqueda, L., Mulnard, R., Liao, S., Gibbs, L., & Fitzgerald, W. (2010). Screening for abuse and neglect of people with dementia. *Journal of the American Geriatrics Society,* 58(3), 493-500. https://doi.org/10.1111/j.1532-5415.2010.02737.x

Wolf, R.S. (1989, June 7). Oral testimony for *Elder abuse: An assessment of the federal response,* Congressional hearing before the Subcommittee on Human Services. Washington, D.C.

World Health Organization. (2020). *Elder abuse.* Retrieved from https://www.who.int/en/news-room/fact-sheets/detail/elder-abuse

Yunus, R.M., Hairi, N.N., & Choo, W.Y. (2019). Consequences of elder abuse and neglect: A systematic review of observational studies. *Trauma, Violence, & Abuse,* 20(2), 197-213. https://doi.org/10.1177/1524838017692798

FIGURE 1: Key Sets of Elder Abuse Policy Recommendations

National Policy Summit on Elder Abuse Final Action Agenda

- Develop and implement a sustained national strategic communications program to educate the public on elder abuse

- Enact a National Elder Abuse Act

- Improve the legal landscape for the justice system

- Fund the development and implementation of a national elder abuse education/training curriculum for use by various professionals

- Expand the availability and accessibility of age-appropriate mental health services

- Commission a Government Accounting Office study of current federal and state expenditures on elder abuse in relationship to service needs

- Increase awareness within the justice system

- Establish a research and program institute within the National Institute on Aging to improve research, data collection, and reporting elder abuse

- Create a national APS resource center

- Seek an Executive Order by the President directing federal agencies and inviting governors to review all policies to better coordinate preventions, interventions, services, and victim assistance for maltreated older adults

(National Center on Elder Abuse, 2002)

The Elder Justice Roadmap First Wave Policy Action Items and Policy Priorities

First Wave Policy Action Items

- Improve law, policies, training, oversight, and data collection related to substituted decision-making

- Build a strong movement to advance elder justice

- Develop national APS definitions and standards

Policy Priorities

- Develop national APS definitions, collaborations, training requirements, data collection mechanism, training, technical assistance, and standards as well as create a national office for APS

- Assess existing programs, laws, and trainings to ensure efficacy and inclusivity when identifying policy priorities and what programs, laws, and trainings to replicate

- Fully fund and implement elder justice provisions in existing federal laws

- Promulgate guidance to assist Institutional Review Boards, researchers, and multidisciplinary teams in navigating consent and other human-subjects protection issues in elder abuse research

- Develop infrastructure to promote consistency, coordination, efficiency, and focus on policy development, practice, research, and training at the federal, state, and local levels

- Strengthen monitoring of long-term care services and supports and examine policies to better prevent, detect, and redress abuse and neglect in home, community-based, and institutional long-term care settings

- Examine how Medicare and Medicaid policy could be modified to prevent and mitigate elder abuse

- Cultivate and fund multidisciplinary efforts in elder abuse matters

- Develop coordinated, well-funded advocacy entities and multidisciplinary networks to inform policy, increase resources, and raise awareness at national, state, and local levels

- Engage in and partner with a variety of overlapping fields whose constituencies are affected by elder abuse

- Identify and develop policy to respond to transitions that might heighten the risk of elder abuse

(Connolly, Brandl, & Breckman, 2014)

FIGURE 2: Elder Abuse Policy Challenges

- Persistent ageism, resulting in diminished interest around issues affecting older adults

- Inadequate data, particularly what might be useful for legislative advocacy

- Competing interests, including from the domestic violence programs community

- Lack of confidence in select existing interventions, such as APS

- Inadequate enforcement of existing laws, illustrated by OBRA 1987

- Few Congressional and state champions

- Insufficient stature of existing advocacy groups, especially in comparison with such other issues as child abuse, with its Children's Defense Fund

- Few Congressional hearings, needed to focus on the issue and discuss legislative provisions

- The image of elder abuse as a private matter

- Powerful lobbies in opposition, particularly those representing long-term care facilities and against consumer protections

- Lack of federal or state coordinating offices

- Scant research, especially on policy matters

- Continuing controversies around select policy provisions, including mandatory reporting and client confidentiality among involved professionals from external agencies

- Uncertainty about the effectiveness of key intervention systems for improving the safety and status of victims rather than causing them further harm

- Lack of belief in existing policy and programming options for perpetrators

- Fear of over regulation, particularly having more imposed on long-term care facilities and services

- Confusing policy definitions and provisions, such as what really constitutes elder abuse and who qualifies for intervention

FIGURE 3: Elder Abuse Policy Opportunities

- Elder abuse is a bipartisan issue that seems equally attractive to both Democrats and Republicans.

- Current concerns about financial abuse have broad appeal, particularly to baby boomers and their families, often faced with potential longevity greater than retirement assets.

- Leadership in the field of elder abuse has been dogged about applying lessons learned from analogous fields.

- Increasing numbers of state and local elder abuse networks can affect important policy change.

- The growth of interagency collaboration at all government levels around addressing elder abuse can foster more integrative policy.

- Reauthorization requirements for various federal elder abuse laws provide the ability to expand, improve, and update provisions.

- Political advocacy across generations can be tapped around a problem that has implications for more than just older adult victims.

- Current news drivers have had the effect of sparking greater political engagement and social activism, some of which can be directed toward the issue of elder abuse.

- The growth of elder abuse research and its improved methodology toward determining sound practice and policy provides essential information toward deciding where advocacy should be directed.

Age-Differentiated vs. Age-Integrated: Neoliberal Policy and the Future of the Life Course

Dale Dannefer, PhD[1*]

Jielu Lin, PhD[2]

George Gonos, PhD[3]

[1] Case Western Reserve University, Department of Sociology

[2] National Insititutes of Health

[3] Florida International University, Center for Labor Research and Studies

*Corresponding Author: dxd79@case.edu

Acknowledgements: The authors wish to thank two anonymous reviewers for critical and constructive comments. We thank Reema Sen for valuable research and editorial assistance.

ABSTRACT

Observing the human costs for persons of all ages of the institutionalized tripartite life course (ILC) characterizing advanced postindustrial societies, gerontological pioneer Matilda White Riley proposed an "age-integrated" alternative that would support a more balanced engagement with education, work, and leisure (i.e., retirement) across the life course. Without denying the kinds of manifest benefits that the ILC has provided to modern citizens (notably enhanced educational opportunities and retirement support), Riley rightly pointed out the opportunities lost due to the restrictions imposed by the normative age-graded or age-differentiated model of the "three-box" life course. However, both the age-segmented ILC and the age-integrated alternative envisioned by Riley have presupposed the broad floor of support of essential components of the life course (i.e., education, work and retirement/leisure) provided by the post-World War II social contract. We demonstrate that this floor of support has been dangerously eroded by the neoliberal turn in social policy, which has undermined that social contract. Ironically, the ideas of a more individualized or "flexible" life course are often co-opted to legitimate the off-loading of risk to individuals that is integral to neoliberal policy. In reality, viable implementation of Riley's proposed age-integrated

doi: 10.18278/jep.1.2.3

model would require a rejection of such policies and a renewed public commitment at least equal to the support that undergirded the institutionalized life course. We detail some dimensions of neo-liberalism's impact on the life course, and we suggest the types of policy changes that could rebuild support for the institution of the life course, with special attention to Riley's age-integrated model and its potential to advance human interests.

Keywords: flexible work schedules, institutionalized life course, social contract, structural lag

Diferenciación por edad vs. integración por edad: Política neoliberal y futuro del curso de vida

Resumen

Al observar los costos humanos para las personas de todas las edades del curso de vida tripartito institucionalizado (ILC) que caracteriza a las sociedades postindustriales avanzadas, la pionera gerontológica Matilda White Riley propuso una alternativa "integrada por edad" que respaldaría un compromiso más equilibrado con la educación, el trabajo y el ocio. (es decir, jubilación) a lo largo de la vida. Sin negar los tipos de beneficios manifiestos que la ILC ha brindado a los ciudadanos modernos (en particular, mejores oportunidades educativas y apoyo a la jubilación), Riley señaló correctamente las oportunidades perdidas debido a las restricciones impuestas por el modelo normativo graduado por edad o diferenciado por edad de la Curso de vida de "tres cajas". Sin embargo, tanto la ILC segmentada por edad como la alternativa integrada por edad imaginada por Riley han supuesto el amplio piso de apoyo de los componentes esenciales del curso de la vida (es decir, educación, trabajo y jubilación / ocio) proporcionado por la posguerra. contrato social. Demostramos que este piso de apoyo ha sido peligrosamente erosionado por el giro neoliberal en la política social, que ha socavado ese contrato social. Irónicamente, las ideas de un curso de vida más individualizado o "flexible" a menudo son cooptadas para legitimar la descarga de riesgo para los individuos que es parte integral de la política neoliberal. En realidad, la implementación viable del modelo integrado por edades propuesto por Riley requeriría un rechazo de tales políticas y un compromiso público renovado al menos igual al apoyo que sustentaba el curso de vida institucionalizado. Detallamos algunas dimensiones del impacto del neoliberalismo en el curso de la vida, y sugerimos los tipos de cambios de política que podrían reconstruir el apoyo a la institución del curso de la vida, con especial atención al modelo integrado por edades de Riley y su potencial para promover los intereses humanos.

Palabras clave: Curso de vida, política neoliberal, modelo integrado por edades

区分年龄VS.整合年龄：新自由主义政策和生命历程的未来

摘要

观察到制度化三段式生命历程（ILC）（高等后工业化社会的典型特征）对各年龄段人群产生的人类成本，老年学先驱者Matilda White Riley提出了一个"整合年龄的"替代方案，该方案支持对生命历程中的教育、工作和娱乐（即退休）进行更均衡的安排。在不否认ILC为现代公民提供的各类显而易见的益处（最重要的是提升教育机会和退休支持）的情况下，Riley正确地指出了因三段式生命历程的规范化年龄分级或年龄区分模式所产生的限制而丢失的机遇。不过，年龄区分型ILC和Riley所设想的年龄整合替代方案都假设二战后建立的社会契约为生命历程的基本部分（即教育、工作和退休/娱乐）提供广泛支持。我们证明，这种支持已被社会政策中的新自由主义转变所严重侵蚀，它损害了这种社会契约。可笑的是，关于一个更个体化或更"灵活"的生命历程的观点如今常被用于对"个体风险的去除"进行合法化，而这种风险是新自由主义政策必不可少的一部分。在现实中，以可行的方式执行Riley的年龄整合模式将要求拒绝这类政策，并需要一个新的公共承诺，这种承诺至少应提供制度化生命历程所需的支持。我们详细描述了新自由主义对生命历程所产生的影响的部分维度，并建议了那些能重建生命历程制度所需支持的政策变革类型，特别聚焦于Riley的年龄整合模式及其在提升人类利益方面的潜能。

关键词：生命历程，新自由主义政策，年龄整合模式 (Age-Integrated Model)

Matilda White Riley, a pioneering founder of the sociology of age and the life course as a field of study, was also herself a model of active aging, continuing to work well past her 90th birthday (see, e.g, Dannefer, Uhlenberg, Foner & Abeles, 2005; Dannefer, Foner & Hess, 2000). Thus, she not only was a leading expert on aging, but herself experienced firsthand the "gains and losses" (Baltes, 1987), the opportunities and challenges that come with age, including the socially imposed challenges associated with ageism and age segregation and discrimination.

A "Functional Failure" of Social Order

Riley was a longtime colleague and close personal friend of both Talcott Parsons and Robert Merton, so it should not be surprising that her approach to sociological analysis was framed by the paradigmatic assumptions of American structural-functionalism, of which Parsons and Merton were primary architects. Structural-functionalism offered a rather upbeat and hopeful narrative of society and social progress that resonated with the economic and educational expansion of the post-WWII period and treated problems such as poverty and racism as aberrations that could surely be solved with continued societal progress, and with just a little more time.

Thus, it is especially telling that Riley's last book, coauthored in 1994 with Anne Foner and psychologist Robert Kahn, was titled *Age and Structural Lag: Society's **Failure** to Provide Mean-* *ingful Opportunities in Work, Family and Leisure* (emphasis ours). The idea of a "societal failure" is quite at odds with Parsonian functionalism, which regards any society that manages to survive and flourish as successful, and in the case of the U.S. and the post-WWII West more generally, as becoming more so all the time (e.g., Parsons, 1972). To call out a "societal failure" within this framework implies that the failure in question must indeed be consequential, and one that requires systematic attention to be redressed. What is this "failure"? It is the societal imposition of restricted, age-graded activity routines that squelch human possibilities:

> [T]he major responsibilities for work and family are still crowded into what are now the middle years of long life, while education is primarily reserved for the young, and leisure and free time are disproportionately allocated to the later years .... Our failure to match in social structures the rapid gains in longevity, health and style of life has had the unintended consequences of creating a poor fit between social institutions and people's capabilities and responsibilities at every age (Riley, Kahn & Foner, 1994, p. 2).

Elaborating the problem further, Riley & Riley note:

> [T]he unprecedented increases in longevity ... mean that people spend one-third of their adult lives in retirement (which) ... consists largely of "unstructured time" ....While young and

middle-aged adults, especially women, are deprived of free time by the doubly demanding roles of work and family, older people tend to be surfeited with it. Yet there are few normative expectations to give meaning to this time or to their lives, and few employment or other opportunities to participate with younger people in the mainstream activities of society (Riley & Riley, 1994, p. 16).

Thus, as a result of increasing longevity, "lives have been drastically altered ... but numerous inflexible social structures, roles and norms have lagged behind" (Riley & Riley, 1994, p. 16). Riley's critical argument is further underscored by the fact that midlife "work" actually includes "the subcontracting of work" from employers to families (Kanter, 1977) and other forms of unpaid domestic labor, the burden of which falls disproportionately on women.

This general situation is what Riley terms "structural lag," which she appraises as a general problem, and one that is especially relevant to the situation of elders: "[S]tructural lag and the need for change are currently most conspicuous for older people, because of their protracted longevity, their increasing numbers in the population, and—save for the disadvantaged minority—their remarkably good health and effective functioning" (1994, p. 18). Similar concerns regarding the potential human costs and counter-productivity of the "three-box" life course has also been expressed by scholars working from other theoretical traditions (e.g., Dannefer,

1989; Phillipson, 2002).

Taking this challenge as a point of departure, this article addresses three interrelated problems concerning the structuring of the life course. The first is to consider the modern life course as a general, socially structured phenomenon that was established in the 20th Century and within it, more specifically, the implications of two contrasting models that Riley counterposed, the "age-differentiated" and "age-integrated" models. The second issue, yet more fundamental, is to examine how the life course as a societal construct and institution has itself come under assault—an assault that encompasses both of these alternative models. Finally, we consider the possibilities for advanced industrial societies to develop and support the personal control and flexibility envisioned in Riley's age-integrated model as we enter the third decade of the new century.

Models of the Life Course: Variations on a Modern Theme

Based on her notion of structural lag and her observations regarding the often-costly strains and restrictions imposed upon the life course by the tripartite "age-differentiated" approach, Riley counterposes to it what she terms an "age-integrated" model of life-course organization (see Figure 1). This straightforward diagram makes explicit the possibility of conceiving education, work and leisure as spread across the life course, rather than occurring in age-segmented, sequential mass doses.

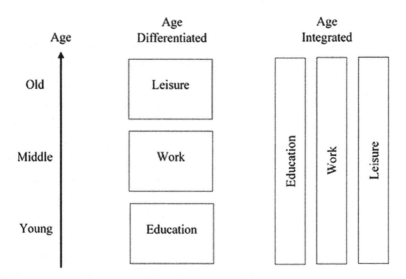

Figure 1. Age-Differentiated and Age-Integrated Models of the Life Course
(from Riley & Riley, 1994, p. 26).

Riley's critique notwithstanding, some social scientists have presented a more positive view of the education/work/retirement sequence that she terms the "age-differentiated" model. In particular, Martin Kohli, who has observed that this model of the life course is so established and integral to the modern social order that it is appropriately considered a social institution, notes its benefits. He suggests that the social institution of the life course is key to solving practical and existential problems for individuals, organizing their lives experientially and biographically, providing economic and social security, and providing some sense of orderliness and even of meaning (Kohli, 2007).

With respect to social policy, it is worth noting that the institutionalized, tripartite life course (ILC) is itself largely the product of deliberate, age-graded policy innovations, including policies establishing mass, free public education and those providing state support for work exit and retirement (via public as well as private pension programs, and in some cases, age-based mandatory retirement). These social innovations have of course been integral to the development of modern forms of social organization and the modern state. They provide the societal framework within which individuals approach later life and have major implications for the nature of experience in old age. Indeed, for advanced industrial societies generally such innovations have arguably contributed importantly to positive changes in the experience of the later years and old age, via the economic benefits of education, and via the reduction of old-age poverty and concomitant improvements in health, longevity and quality of life in the later years. These are palpable benefits of the life course as a social institution.

Yet despite such benefits, Riley's critique makes clear that the "three-box" age-differentiated paradigm is not without its own very substantial problems. In addition to the costs she recounts at the level of individual experience, the age-based segmentation of experience is also responsible for numerous demographic strains. At the base of the tripartite organization of the life course can be laid some of the most pressing social and economic challenges faced by advanced postindustrial societies, notably the old-age dependency ratio (Hammer, Prskawetz & Freund, 2015; Ingham, Chirijevskis & Carmichael, 2009) and strains placed on age-graded education (Gradstein & Kaganovich, 2004) and on work, healthcare, and other institutions as disparately sized cohorts make their way through the life course (Anderson & Hussey, 2000; Uhlenberg, 1992). The much-debated "generation wars" stoked by advocates of "Generational Equity" and related movements, are also predicated on the assumption of a tripartite division and the back-loading of years of leisure (see, e.g., Quadagno, 1989; Walker, 2013). Similarly, the tripartite structure has been an essential premise for arguments used to justify Social Security privatization (e.g., that claiming the shorter life expectancy of black persons meant that privatization would benefit them [see Tanner, 2001]).

Beyond such macro-level considerations, other scholars have, consistent with Riley's concerns, analyzed the psychologically and relationally adverse consequences of social arrangements that encourage and sustain age-segregated patterns of social interaction in the life course (e.g., Hagestad & Uhlenberg, 2005; 2006).

Especially in professional human services domains such as counseling and human development, the human costs of the "three-box" life course and the promise of a more open and less scripted approach to aging had received considerable attention, even before the time of Riley's writing (e.g., Best, 1980, Bolles, 1978; Neugarten, 1968; Sarason, 1977; Whitbourne, 1985). Increasingly, through the 1970s and 1980s, the oppressiveness of rigid age-graded expectations became an existential preoccupation.

Related to this tension between the age-differentiated and age-integrated models, Riley and associates (1994, p. 3) detail a range of policy issues and questions prompted by the problem of structural lag, which were being discussed at the time of their writing. These include:

- Whether to spread work more evenly over the life course, by providing longer vacations, flexible work hours, incentives for midlife switching to new careers

- Whether to reduce heavy transfer payments by the middle aged and to require that both the old and the young become more self-supporting

- How to determine the appropriate age for retirement

- How to design communities, housing, shopping centers, roadways to meet human needs that are changing over the life course.

Such critique and such questions notwithstanding, when viewed in historical perspective, the institutionalized age-differentiated life course clearly represented an advance over what came before. It provided many citizens with universal K-12 schooling and expanding educational opportunities, stable employment and, after the working years, economically supported free time. It must be kept in mind that such benefits did not extend in the same form to all segments of the population; African-Americans and other minorities were in many ways deliberately shortchanged (see, e.g., Poole, 2006). Yet compared to the more unpredictable, contingent and often precarious biographical patterns that preceded it (see, e.g, Achenbaum, 1978; 2009; Chudacoff, 1989; Kett, 1977), it provided stability, coherence and even existential meaning to the experience of aging, arguably with great benefit, even for many disadvantaged minorities (Katznelson, 2005: Kohli, 2007). Yet Riley contended that this tripartite, age-graded configuration does not represent the last word on the subject, any more than the automobiles and aircraft of the mid-20th century were the last word in transportation technology. Riley and colleagues offer a progressive view that builds on the premise of a publicly supported floor of security and enhances human prospects.

Few would deny the appeal of Riley's age-integrated model. For example, removing age-based restrictions to participating in work could offer greater control to individuals while also contributing to societal productivity and welfare (Uhlenberg, 1988; 1996), and providing more support for midlife education or specialized training could enhance human capital and productivity. However, the use of policy to provide support for a more flexibly configured life course, relying less on chronological age as an organizing criterion, has yet to be pursued beyond a few fragmentary initiatives (e.g., *Bildungsurlaub* in Germany, or in Austria, or "career break" policies in Belgium and other EU countries or "time credit" systems [Phillipson, 2002, p. 24]). Given the potential advantages of the age-integrated life course, the dearth of attention to policy initiatives that would provide support for age-integrated alternatives in the U.S. is unfortunate. While the elimination of mandatory retirement does comprise an important step in such a direction for older citizens, that step does nothing to support any form of educational or other life-course innovation for those in the middle years. It also does nothing to provide support for older persons who may have worked hard all their lives yet are economically compelled to continue working (Burkert & Hochfellner, 2017). Thus, it may be seen as a mixed blessing. At a conference panel in the 1990s, representatives of the AARP and the union-based National Council of Senior Citizens (NCSC) were each asked to identify the most significant advance in U.S. ageing policy. For the AARP, it was "eliminating mandatory retirement"; for the NCSC, it was "lowering the retirement age to 62" (Hudson, 2012; see also Phillipson, 2002). As Rob Hudson noted in relaying this exchange, when you have spent your days slapping hubcaps on Chevies, "mandatory retirement" is no threat; it is more likely welcomed. In fact, however, the share of people 65 and older who are employed is now higher than in over half a century (Morrissey, 2016).

The Life Course as an Institution: Tensions and Possibilities

Although it would be heartening to see more public discussion and support for such issues, more immediate challenges that confront the very notion of the life-course construct as a modern institution must be addressed. Indeed, over the past several decades the very idea of the life course as a general, public provision of biographical stability and support has come under assault, so that both sides of the debate face a common threat of an erosion of commitment to the economic viability of the key premises and components of life-course security.

This assault can be seen in the constant rhetoric that retirement, age-graded or not, can no longer be "afforded," as some corporate and political leaders have maintained (e.g., Petersen, 1999), creating pressure to increase retirement age and reduce pension benefits (Phillipson, 2002). In the USA and elsewhere, it is also evident in the breach of promised pensions and in the shift from defined benefits to defined contributions (Quadagno & Street, 2006). The shift from traditional defined-benefit pensions to retirement savings accounts (defined contribution plans) has widened retirement disparities. In

2013, nearly nine in 10 families in the top income quintile had retirement account savings, compared with fewer than one in 10 families in the bottom income quintile. Most families in the bottom half of the income distribution have no retirement account savings at all (e.g., Russell, 2014; Morrissey, 2016). One effect of these changes can be seen in the growth of inequality and precarity among older persons (Crystal et al., 2017; Phillipson, 2013; Shuey & O'Rand 2004; Weller & Newman, 2020), made palpable by their visible presence as Wal-Mart greeters and grocery-store baggers. Declining support for the life course is no less evident early in the life course, where funding for public education has been ratcheted down in recent years (Leachman, Masterson & Figueroa, 2017), and where student loan debt is daunting if not disastrous for young adults trying to launch a career.

This constellation of assaults has affected the immediate practical viability both of the "age-differentiated" institutionalized life course and of the possibility of implementing Riley's "age-integrated" alternative, because both of these approaches—despite their differences—share a crucially important, common premise. This premise is the existence of a sturdy floor of social and economic support for the lives of individual citizens, which renders possible the idea of a reasonable level of general social stability and economic security as a context for planning a biography, or at least the next steps in it.

The premise of a stable foundation for individual economic survival seemed well established at the time the age-integrated life course was first articulated in the 1970s. Especially during the quarter century from 1947 to 1973, in the wake of the New Deal and riding the tide of postwar prosperity, a heightened sense of the possibilities of orderly and predictable life planning was increasingly undergirded by a strong labor market, and by the assumption that those "glory days" of the post-World War II U.S. social contract would remain in place (Bluestone & Bluestone,1992). The reality of a coherent, largely scripted biography following the age-differentiated model was facilitated by a broad array of intersecting institutions—private as well as public.

It is important to understand how institutions and policies in the post-World War II period were customized to support the institutionalization of the life course. Importantly, the age-differentiated life course trajectory was undergirded by internal labor markets (ILMs) in the workplace. ILMs represented a trade-off. In exchange for the employer's offer of long-term job security, employees agreed to sacrifice a portion of their earned wages during the early phases of their tenure in exchange for the promise of a stable, decent retirement after a prolonged period (typically 30 years) of service—in the form of the (now nearly-extinct) defined-benefit retirement pensions. Along the way, workers were incentivized to remain productive by the employer's provision of training, rising wages and benefits, and regular promotion opportunities (Stone, 2004, p. 51-63; Adams & Heywood, 2007; Zwick, 2012). During this period, moreover, wages were steadily

increasing and federal legislation supported a standard 40-hour work week, which assisted workers in maintaining a modicum of family life.

In addition to the ILM, state policies, including the GI Bill and Social Security, offered (to white citizens, at least) a high level of public investment in young adulthood in the form of support for college education and homeowner loans, as well as a floor of financial protection against the hazards in later life. In short, economic prosperity, combined with specific public policies, created the institutional uniformity of age-differentiated life course trajectories.

But while ILMs could make the retirement years materially comfortable, they also carried additional adverse consequences that would later become the focus of Riley's and other critiques of the ILC. Before reaching retirement, blue-collar workers faced the cumulative disadvantage of long years of often deadening and debilitating work (Hayward, Friedman & Chen, 1996; Kelly, 2000; Marucci-Wellman, Willetts, Lin, Brennan & Verma, 2014; Neff, 1985). And given the lack of a valued role for retirees in the age-differentiated model, blue- and white-collar workers alike often experienced less than fully satisfying lives in their senior years. Moreover, as is becoming increasingly well known, the benefits of many of these aspects of the social contract, including Social Security, retirement pensions, college tuition benefits, and homeowner loans, were never extended to all segments. Minorities, women, those without jobs in the "core" economy, and many segments of the young and old populations, were conspicuously excluded (Dannefer, Gilbert & Han, 2020; Katznelson, 2005; Rothstein, 2017). The relative stability and material comfort in retirement were in many cases not conferred upon members of those groups.

Despite such significant shortcomings, the institutionalized life course nevertheless provided, as Martin Kohli emphasizes, an expanding base of economic security and a sense of biographical predictability that anchored work, family and personal life for large segments of the population and, for better or worse, created a defined public narrative of the life course. Although the issue of inclusion/exclusion remained to be adequately addressed (Kohli, 2008), the ILC represented an arrangement that scores of millions of workers and families eagerly embraced, depicted with everyday descriptors like "company man" or "set up for life."

Neoliberalism and the Collapse of the Institutionalized Life Course

In the late 1970s, the rising dominance of neoliberal policies began to undermine the floor of social and economic support that had made the age-differentiated life course possible. At the core of neoliberalism is a stated belief in free markets as a guide to policy. Under its influence, governments have championed the deregulation of business, and of labor and financial markets, the privatization of public services, steep reductions in tax-es, and cuts in social welfare programs (Harvey, 2005; Saad-Filho & Johnston, 2005).

Launched by shifts in political leadership and policy in the U.S., Britain, and China, the impact of neoliberalism was not long in coming. Neoliberal policies entailed a reduced commitment to the broad-based, publicly supported social contract across the central domains of education, work life, and retirement that had been expanded over prior decades. For many individuals and families, the premises of individual economic security and social stability that provided the foundation of the life course as a socially supported institution began to erode palpably. The "glory days" of well-paying and seemingly secure industrial and corporate jobs receded with surprising rapidity, replaced by uncertainty and anxiety (Bluestone & Bluestone, 1992, p. 60-106; Standing, 2011). With neoliberal ideologies justifying the subjugation of citizen welfare to corporate competitiveness, citizens became preoccupied with the precarity of life-course security.

A concomitant of this change of direction can be seen in the sharp upward redistribution of the nation's income occurring through the same time period. One indication is displayed in Figure 2, which traces the relationship between productivity and wages since 1948. As can be clearly seen, the wages of nonsupervisory workers grew in tandem with productivity until the mid-1970s, after which point wages flattened. The result, as economists at the Economic Policy Institute conclude, is "an overall shift in how much of the income in the economy is received by workers in wages and benefits, and how much is received by owners." Thus, as they further explain, "[R]ising productivity in recent decades provided the *potential for a substantial growth in the pay for the vast majority of workers*" (Bivens & Mishel, 2015, our emphasis). However, "this potential was squandered," as nearly all of the added value generated by increased productivity went to corporate owners, rather than workers, fueling the growth of extreme inequality.

Figure 2 makes clear that these two measures tracked closely until the mid 1970s, when wage growth leveled off, creating a growing, long-term divergence. A comprehensive analysis of the factors accounting for this divergence lie beyond the scope of this paper. However, one significant set of such factors responsible for this pattern derives from pressures to reduce labor costs and regulatory oversight, which led to the mass exportation of manufacturing and other jobs from the U.S. and other advanced societies. This practice not only cost millions of jobs, but also created downward wage pressure on domestic workers, and weakened unions. Jack Welch, the celebrated CEO of General Electric from 1981 to 2001, epitomized this logic when he described as a corporate ideal, "...having every plant you own on a barge" (Palley, 2007) that could quickly relocate to wherever a new source of cheap labor might be found—a telling vision of the implications of the logic of capital for anything like a social contract, and of the global "race to the bottom" for workers' pay.

To put this productivity-wage gap in perspective, it is also instructive to give further consideration to the slice of the economic pie paid to workers. Our analysis (available on request) of data from the Bureau of Labor Statistics shows that the total economic output for the U.S. in 1970 was just over 2 trillion (in current dollars), with 62% of that (1.28 trillion) paid to workers. By 2018 the output had increased almost 8-fold to 15.68 trillion (in current dollars), with a *decrease* in labor share to 56%, or 8.86 trillion. Had the share of compensation kept pace with post-WWII level, at 65%, from 1979 to 2018 a total of 18.1 trillion could have gone to members of the workforce—more than double the amount they actually received.

Parallel to this dramatic divergence, or "U-Turn," in Harrison and Bluestone's terms, consider trends of income inequality over this same time period. As can be seen in Figure 3, the mid-1970s also mark a turning point in the distribution of national income, with the share of pre-tax national income going to the bottom 50% of the population decreasing dramatically (from 20% to 12% of the total) while the share of the top 1% increased by roughly the same amount. Thus, these two groups—the bottom 50% and the top 1%— essentially traded places in their share of the income distribution.

These data on productivity, wages and inequality arguably reveal some of the factors involved in the erosion of an economically secure, structural-

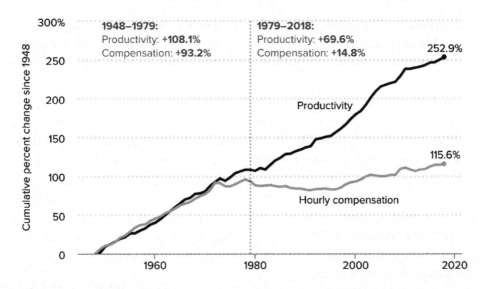

Notes: Data are for compensation (wages and benefits) of production/nonsupervisory workers in the private sector and net productivity of the total economy. "Net productivity" is the growth of output of goods and services less depreciation per hour worked.

Source: EPI analysis of unpublished Total Economy Productivity data from Bureau of Labor Statistics (BLS) Labor Productivity and Costs program, wage data from the BLS Current Employment Statistics, BLS Employment Cost Trends, BLS Consumer Price Index, and Bureau of Economic Analysis National Income and Product Accounts

Updated from Figure A in *Raising America's Pay: Why It's Our Central Economic Policy Challenge* (Bivens et al. 2014)

Figure 2. Productivity Growth and Hourly Compensation Growth, 1948-2018 (Economic Policy Institute)

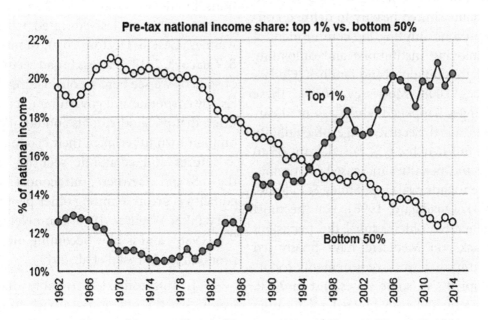

Figure 3. National Income Share of Bottom 50% and Top 1%, Usa 1962-2014 (Piketty, Saez & Zucman, 2016)

ly and publicly supported life-course regime. The expansion of neoliberal policies severely reduced support for the programs that had established the institutionalized life course and has undermined the prospects for a sense of biographical security that the institutionalized life course provided, while contributing to a growing economic precarity faced by large segments of the midlife and older populations, as well as by young people (Standing, 2011). Together they give a sense of the immense wealth lost to workers and their families after 1975 as they tried to plan their lives according to the script provided by the ILC.

The decline in wages is, of course, not the only form of decline in both private and public resources to individuals and families. Some longstanding corporate pension funds either imploded or scaled back benefits and as noted earlier, employers offering defined pension benefits shifted heavily to defined contributions, limiting the commitment of employing institutions and offloading risk to individuals and families (Ghilarducci, 2008; Morrissey, 2016). These changes happened while, as noted earlier, Social Security's age of eligibility for full benefits was raised from 65 to 67, and penalties increased for premature withdrawals (see Shuey & O'Rand, 2004; Quadagno, 1996). For the most vulnerable older adults, the persistent attacks on Medicaid have finally led to imposed work requirements for its recipients in some states and in 2020, allowing states to cap federal funding into the program. The same neoliberal assaults were evident at the beginning

of the life course, in reductions in support for K-12 public education and higher education. Today, roughly 70% of American students end up taking out loans to go to college. This reduction is arguably a significant contributor to the cost of higher education and to the student debt crisis (Hartlep, Eckrich & Hensley, 2017). The average graduate leaves school with around $30,000 in debt and all told, some 45 million Americans owe $1.6 trillion in student loans—and counting (Fields, 2019).

The broad impact of such changes has not been distributed evenly across different sectors of the population. This is evident in the dramatic rise in precarity—in the rapid increase in individuals having to work multiple jobs, in the continuing growth of trajectories of income inequality in each succeeding cohort (Piketty, Saez & Guzman, 2016; Crystal et al., 2017), and in the reductions in life expectancy for key subgroups, including less-educated white women (Case & Deaton, 2020; Montez & Zajacova, 2014). Across broad sectors of society, we see here an off-loading of risk by corporate and governmental entities, that puts individuals and families on their own in terms of their economic futures and economic security. In the U.S. and elsewhere, intracohort inequality is greatest among older people (Crystal & Waehrer, 1996; Dannefer & Sell, 1988), and is now becoming more pronounced (Crystal et al., 2017).

In this context, it is more than ironic that the offloading of risk from public and corporate entities to individuals and families has sought legitimacy by co-opting some of the elements advanced by the "age-integrated model" for neoliberalism's own ideological purposes. Those who advocate reducing or eliminating the benefits of the institutionalized life course will understandably utilize any notions of "free agency" to justify the breakdown of its structures and legitimate the growth of midlife precarity. Thus, students and young employees are now regularly informed that the "restrictive" one-career life is over, and that they will have the "opportunity" to develop a "flexible," "do-it-yourself" career (e.g., Kunda, 1992, p. 122-125). Such impulses have multiple parallels across disparate kinds of work settings, as when truckers are encouraged to become owner-operator truckers, "owning" their truck (mortgaged to a bank of course) and assuming all the risks of its value, insurance, repairs, and upkeep (Black, 2009; Smith, Bensman & Marvy, 2010), or when functions traditionally handled in-house are outsourced to employees misclassified as "independent contractors" who typically work without the integral provision of any pension, healthcare or other such benefits. The spread of contingent labor throughout the economy has increased precarity and undermined the feasibility of life planning at every stage of the life course (Barker & Christensen, 1998; Hatton, 2011; Gonos & Martino, 2011).

Similarly, in the domain of retirement pensions, a dominant narrative claimed that it would be a "good deal" and "great opportunity" to switch from defined benefit to defined contribution retirement plans (e.g., Gustman & Steinmeier, 1999; Kotlikoff, 1996;

Russell, 2014). All such efforts represent ideologies to provide legitimation for the growth of midlife precarity.

Such precarity is a far cry from what Riley and others have had in mind with the conception of a flexible, age-integrated life course, which rests on the floor of the social contract and in which flexibility is primarily under the control of the aging person, not the employer who promotes "flexibilization" to put employees on standby (see Phillipson, 2002). Riley envisioned a cultural shift in which the idea for meaningful, life-long productivity allowed for greater individual control and autonomy. However, such a shift would necessarily presuppose continuity with the social contract of the institutionalized life course, with broad social and institutional support, and strong societal purchase and warrant.

Protecting the Experience of Aging: Policy Directions to Rebuild the Life Course

The growing precarity associated with the decline of a socially supported life course regime clearly has implications for health and quality of life as individuals move through the life course and into old age. It is important to remember that the life course regime was originally organized by social policies, and its decline can be attributed at least partially to policy changes (e.g., reducing support for basic and advanced education; drastic reductions in the tax rate on high income earners from the 1960s to the present; reduced retirement options and benefits). While such policies do not necessarily bear directly on old age, they do have implications for midlife earnings and related benefits—factors which, in turn, predict a great deal about late-life health and quality of life. For gerontologists, to be unconcerned with such issues is to be unconcerned with how equipped coming generations of elders are as they enter later life and old age.

While this is not the place to undertake a comprehensive analysis of potentially relevant policy initiatives, the foregoing analysis makes clear that at least one domain that warrants attention is the domain of earnings, and specifically the need to reestablish the connection between wages and productivity, that obtained prior to the ascent of neoliberal tax and regulatory policies. A wide range of such policy discussions are underway, including a UBI (universal basic income), baby bond proposals, living wage requirements, progressive tax policies, and free college education. As we learn more about the resilience and robustness of the socioeconomic gradient, the implications of such policies for aging and later life can be ignored only at gerontology's peril.

The analysis of productivity presented earlier also points to a second set of circumstances and issues that are perhaps more closely attuned to the specific vision of Riley's model of the age-integrated life course. Such issues include the fact that productivity has continued to increase, quite linearly, since WWII. By definition, when productivity grows, the actual value of an hour of work increases. If workers saw the benefit of

this increase in their wages, they would be in a position to exercise more control over the biographical contours of their own lives. Similarly, restoring more progressive tax policies in the U.S. could help enable adequate health and education to support an age-integrated life course. Greater earnings, and potentially greater savings, could lay the foundation for addressing the excessive midlife demands chronicled by Riley. Such demands have expanded since she wrote about the increasing number of individuals working two jobs, along with the numbers of midlife and aging adults, especially women, compelled to balance work and caregiving demands, or being unable to afford retirement. Put differently, a potential benefit of a fairer distribution of the benefits of increased productivity is that it could enable midlife earners to a) spend more time with family members and other socially rewarding informal activity, b) plan or obtain training for a different occupation or career; and/or c) pursue enriching avocational goals.

In the U.S., the establishment of the 40-hour work week required decades of labor struggle to overcome the staunch resistance and brutal repression of employers who billed the proposal as unaffordable, unworkable, and "revolutionary" (Roediger & Foner, 1989). It wasn't until 1938, when legislation mandated "overtime" pay, along with a "minimum" wage, that the standard 40-hour week became public policy. This norm was an integral part of the life course paradigm that drove postwar prosperity. However, much like other chronometrically-based criteria in society (Chudacoff, 1992; Rogoff, 2003), the conception of a 40-hour work week was incidental, certainly not based on anything in human nature or the science of efficiency. Federal policies for overtime pay and a minimum wage led to the effective normalization of the 40-hour work week. Just as that policy innovation was attacked as an economic impossibility, it is now arguably well past time to explore the implementation of both a "living wage" policy (see Marshall, 2019; Luce, 2004) and further reductions in the normative work week, especially in view of the dramatic productivity gains made possible by technology.

Indeed, if we are to represent the interests of individuals approaching old age during an extended historical period of rising labor productivity, should gerontology not be pointing to the need to explore the feasibility and benefits of, say, a 28- or 30- hour week?[1] This would of course not preclude a longer work week for those who receive intrinsic rewards from their work any more than

do current work-week expectations, but it would be an integral part of a supportive framework to allow those who would relish more control over the finite number of hours in their fast-fleeting lives. This is certainly applicable for those whose work-life offers little rewards or physical assaults on the body, as noted earlier.

One of the now-well-established principles of positive mental health is the importance of having a sense of control over one's life (Heckhausen, 1997; Kahana, Kahana & Lee, 2014; Mirowsky & Ross, 2003). As is now well understood, solid mental and physical health in early life, midlife and throughout the life course are of key importance as a foundation for dealing with the challenges of later life. Thus, a concern with supporting the life course and in particular, supporting developments that can enhance the possibilities for a socially supported yet flexible "age-integrated" life course are key elements in a holistic approach to aging and old age.

References

Achenbaum, A. (1978). *Old age in the new land: The American experience since 1970.* Johns Hopkins Press. http://doi.org/10.1353/book.72152

Achenbaum, W. A. (2009). A history of productive aging and the boomers. In R.B. Hudson (Ed.) *Boomer bust?* (pp. 48-65). Greenwood Press.

Adams, S. J., & Heywood, J. S. (2007). The age of hiring and deferred compensation: evidence from Australia. *Economic Record, 83*(261), 174-190. https://doi.org/10.1111/j.1475-4932.2007.00392.x

Anderson, G. F., & Hussey, P. S. (2000). Population aging: a comparison among industrialized countries. *Health Affairs, 19*(3), 191-203. https://doi.

org/10.1377/hlthaff.19.3.191

Baltes, P. B. (1987). Theoretical propositions of life-span developmental psychology: On the dynamics between growth and decline. *Developmental Psychology, 23*(5), 611.

Barker, K., & Christensen, K. (Eds.). (1998). *Contingent work: American employment relations in transition.* Cornell University Press.

Best, F. (1980). *Flexible life scheduling: Breaking the education-work-retirement lockstep.* Praeger Publishers.

Bivens, J., & Mishel, L. (2015, Sep 2). Understanding the historic divergence between productivity and a typical worker's pay: Why it matters and why it's real. Retrieved from https://www.epi.org/publication/understanding-the-historic-divergence-between-productivity-and-a-typical-workers-pay-why-it-matters-and-why-its-real/

Black, T. (2009). *When a heart turns rock solid: The lives of three Puerto Rican brothers on and off the streets.* Pantheon.

Bluestone, B., & Bluestone, I. (1992). *Negotiating the future: A labor perspective on American business.* Basic Books.

Bolles, R. N. (1978). *Three boxes of life.* Ten Speed Press.

Burkert, C., & Hochfellner, D. (2017). Employment trajectories beyond retirement. *Journal of Aging & Social Policy, 29*(2), 143-167.

Case, A., & Deaton, A. (2020). *Deaths of Despair and the Future of Capitalism.* Princeton University Press.

Chudacoff, H. P. 1989 (1992). *How old are you? Age consciousness in American culture.* Princeton University Press.

Crystal, S., & Waehrer, K. (1996). Later-life economic inequality in longitudinal perspective. *The Journals of Gerontology Series B: Psychological Sciences and Social Sciences, 51*(6), S307-S318.

Crystal, S., Shea, D. G., & Reyes, A. M. (2017). Cumulative advantage, cumulative disadvantage, and evolving patterns of late-life inequality. *The Gerontologist, 57*(5), 910-920.

Dannefer, D. (1989). Human action and its place in theories of aging. *Journal of Aging Studies, 3*(1), 1-20.

Dannefer, D., & Sell, R. R. (1988). Age structure, the life course and" aged heterogeneity": prospects for research and theory. *Comprehensive Gerontology. Section B, Behavioural, Social, and Applied Sciences, 2*(1), 1-10.

Dannefer, D., Uhlenberg, P., Foner, A., & Abeles, R. P. (2005). On the shoulders of a giant: The legacy of Matilda White Riley for gerontology. *The Journals of Gerontology Series B: Psychological Sciences and Social Sciences, 60*(6), S296-S304.

Dannefer, D., Gilbert M., & Han C. (2020). With the Wind at Their Backs: Racism and the Amplification of Cumulative Dis/Advantage. In J.A. Kelley (Ed), *Annual Review of Gerontology and Geriatrics Inequality in Later Life*. 40(1): Springer.

Dannefer, D., Foner, A. & Hess, B. (2000). Matilda White Riley: Teacher and Scholar for All Seasons. *Contemporary Gerontology, 6*(1-3). 72-74

Elwell, C. K. 2014. *Inflation and the Real Minimum Wage: A Fact Sheet*. Washington, DC: Congressional Research Service.

Field, J., Burke, R. J., & Cooper, C. L. (Eds.). (2013). *The Sage handbook of aging, work and society*. Sage. http://dx.doi.org/10.4135/9781446269916

Fields, S (2020, Sep 30) 70% of college students graduate with debt. How did we get here? Marketplace, NPR, Retrieved from https://www.marketplace.org/2019/09/30/70-of-college-students-graduate-with-debt-how-did-we-get-here/

Ghilarducci, T. (2008). *When I'm Sixty-Four*. Princeton University Press. https://doi.org/10.1515/9781400824380

Gonos, G., & Martino, C. (2011). Temp agency workers in New Jersey's logistics hub: The case for a union hiring hall. *WorkingUSA, 14*(4), 499-525. https://doi.org/10.1111/j.1743-4580.2011.00359.x

Gradstein, M., & Kaganovich, M. (2004). Aging population and education finance. *Journal of Public Economics, 88*(12), 2469–2485. https://doi.org/10.1016/s0047-2727(03)00065-3

Gustman, A. L., & Steinmeier, T. L. (1999). What people don't know about their pensions and Social Security: An analysis using linked data from the Health and Retirement Study (No. w7368). National Bureau of Economic Research. Retrieved from https://econpapers.repec.org/scripts/redir.pf?u=http%3A%2F%2Fwww.nber.org%2Fpapers%2Fw7368.pdf;h=repec:nbr:nberwo:7368

Hagestad, G. O., & Uhlenberg, P. (2005). The Social Separation of Old and Young: A Root of Ageism. *Journal of Social Issues, 61*(2), 343–360. https://doi.org/10.1111/j.1540-4560.2005.00409.x

Hagestad, G. O., & Uhlenberg, P. (2006). Should we be concerned about age segregation? *Research on Aging, 28*(6), 638–653. https://doi.org/10.1177/0164 027506291872

Hammer, B., Prskawetz, A., & Freund, I. (2015). Production activities and economic dependency by age and gender in Europe: A cross-country comparison. *Journal of the Economics of Ageing, 5*, 86–97. PubMed. https://doi.org/10.1016/j.jeoa.2014.09.007

Harrison, B., & Bluestone, B. (1990). *The great U-turn: Corporate restructuring and the polarizing of America.* Basic Books.

Hartlep, N. D., Eckrich, L. L., & Hensley, B. O. (Eds.). (2017). *The Neoliberal Agenda and the Student Debt Crisis in US Higher Education: Indebted Collegians of the Neoliberal American University.* Taylor & Francis.

Harvey, D. (2005). *A Brief History of Neoliberalism.* Oxford University Press.

Hatton, E. (2011). *The temp economy: From Kelly girls to permatemps in postwar America.* Temple University Press.

Hayward, M. D., Friedman, S., & Chen, H. (1996). Race inequities in men's retirement. *The Journals of Gerontology Series B: Psychological Sciences and Social Sciences, 51*(1), S1-S10.

Heckhausen, J. (1997). Developmental regulation across adulthood: Primary and secondary control of age-related challenges. *Developmental Psychology, 33*(1), 76–187. https://doi.org/10.1037/0012-1649.33.1.176

Hudson, R. (2012). From Approaches to arrivals: Linking policy to practice in aging. 50th Anniversary Conference of the Benjamin Rose Institute on Aging. Cleveland, OH.

Ingham, B., Chirijevskis, A., & Carmichael, F. (2009). Implications of an increasing old-age dependency ratio: The UK and Latvian experiences compared. *Pensions: An International Journal, 14*(4), 221–230. https://doi.org/10.1057/pm.2009.16

Kahana, E., Kahana, B., & Lee, J. E. (2014). Proactive approaches to successful aging: One clear path through the forest. *Gerontology, 60*(5), 466-474

Kanter, R. M., (1977). *Men and women of the corporation.* Basic Books.

Katz, S. (2005). *Cultural aging. Life Course, Lifestyle and Senior Worlds.* University of Toronto Press, Higher Education Division

Katznelson, I. (2005). *When affirmative action was white: An untold history of racial inequality in twentieth-century America.* WW Norton & Company.

Kelly, G. M. (2000). Employment and concepts of work in the new global economy.

International Labour Review, 139(1), 5–32. https://doi.org/10.1111/j.1564-913x.2000.tb00400.x

Kett, J. (1977). *Rites of passage: Adolescence in America 1790 to the present.* Basic Books.

Kohli, M. (2007): The institutionalization of the life course: Looking back to look ahead. *Research in Human Development, 4*(3-4), 253-271.

Kotlikoff, L. J. (1996). Privatizing social security at home and abroad. *The American Economic Review,* 86(2), 368-372.

Kunda, G. (1992). *Engineering culture: control and commitment in a high-tech corporation.* Temple University Press.

Leachman, M., Masterson, K., & Figueroa, E. (2017). A punishing decade for school funding. Center on Budget and Policy Priorities, 29. Retrieved from https://www.cbpp.org/research/state-budget-and-tax/a-punishing-decade-for-school-funding

Luce, S. 2004. Fighting for a Living Wage. Ithaca, NY: Cornell University Press.

Marucci-Wellman, H. R., Willetts, J. L., Lin, T. C., Brennan, M. J., & Verma, S. K. (2014). Work in multiple jobs and the risk of injury in the US working population. *American Journal of Public Health,* 104(1), 134-142.

Marshall, B. L., & Katz, S. (2012). The embodied life course: Post-ageism or the renaturalization of gender?. *Societies,* 2(4), 222-234

Marshall, S. 2019. Living Wage: Regulatory Solutions to Informal and Precarious Work in Global Supply Chains. Oxford University Press.

Mirowsky, J., & Ross, C. E. (2003). *Education, social status, and health.* Transaction Publishers.

Morrissey, M. (2016). The state of American retirement: How 401 (k) s have failed most American workers. Economic Policy Institute, 3.

Montez, J. K., & Zajacova, A. (2014). Why is life expectancy declining among low-educated women in the United States?. *American Journal of Public Health, 104*(10), e5-e7.

Neff, W. (1985). *Work and Human Behavior.* Routledge.

Neugarten, B. L. (Ed.). (1968). *Middle age and aging.* University of Chicago Press.

Palley, T. I. (2007). Jack Welch's barge: the new economics of trade. Retrieved from http://thomaspalley.com/?p=87

Parsons, T. (1972). *The System of Modern Societies.* Practice-Hall. Inc. Englewood Cliffs.

Peterson, P. (1999). *Grey Dawn.* Random House.

Phillipson, C. (2002). *Transitions from work to retirement: Developing a new social contract.* Policy Press.

Phillipson, C., Field, J., Burke, R., & Cooper, C. (2013). Reconstructing work and retirement: labour market trends and policy issues. *The Sage Handbook of Ageing, Work and Society,* London: Sage, pp. 445-60.

Piketty, T., Saez, E., & Zucman, G. (2016). Distributional National Accounts: Methods and Estimates for the United States (Working Paper No. 22945; Working Paper Series). National Bureau of Economic Research. https://doi.org/10.3386/w22945

Poole, M. (2006). *The segregated origins of social security: African Americans and the welfare state.* Chapel Hill, NC: University of North Carolina Press.

Quadagno, J. (1989). Generational equity and the politics of the welfare state. *Politics & Society, 17*(3), 353-376.

Quadagno, J. (1996). Social security and the myth of the entitlement "Crisis". *The Gerontologist, 36*(3), 391-399.

Quadagno, J., & Street, D. (2006). Recent trends in US social welfare policy: minor retrenchment or major transformation?. *Research on Aging, 28*(3), 303-316.

Riley, M. W., Kahn, R. L., Foner, A., & Mack, K. A. (Eds.). (1994). *Age and structural lag: Society's failure to provide meaningful opportunities in work, family, and leisure.* John Wiley & Sons.

Riley, M. W., & Riley Jr, J. W. (1994). Age integration and the lives of older people. *The Gerontologist, 34*(1), 110-115.

Roediger, D. R., & Foner, P. S. (1989). *Our own time: A history of American labor and the working day.* Verso.

Rogoff, B. (2003). *The cultural nature of human development.* Oxford University Press

Rothstein, R. (2017). *The color of law: A forgotten history of how our government segregated America.* Liveright Publishing.

Russell, J. W. (2014). *Social Insecurity: 401 (k) s and the Retirement Crisis.* Beacon Press.

Saad Filho, A., & Johnston, D. (2005). *Neoliberalism: A critical reader.* University of Chicago Press.

Sarason, S. B. (1977). *Work, aging, and social change: Professionals and the one life-one career imperative.* Free Press.

Shuey, K. M., & O'Rand, A. M. (2004). New risks for workers: Pensions, labor markets, and gender. *Annual Review of Sociology, 30,* 453-477.

Smith, R., Bensman, D., & Marvy, P. A. (2010). The big rig: Poverty, pollution, and the misclassification of truck drivers at America's ports. National Employment Law Project, The union federation Change to Win, and Rutgers University. Retrieved from https://teamster.org/wp-content/uploads/2018/12/povertypollutionandmisclassification.pdf

Standing, G. (2011). *The Precariat: The New Dangerous Class.* Bloomsbury Academic

Standing, G. (2014). *A precariat charter: From denizens to citizens.* A&C Black.

Stone, K. V. W. (2004). *From Widgets to Digits.* Cambridge University Press. https://doi.org/10.1017/cbo9780511617089

Tanner, M.D. (2001, Feb 5) The African American Stake in Social Security Reform. Cato Institute. Retrieved from https://www.cato.org/publications/commentary/african-american-stake-social-security-reform

Uhlenberg, P. (1988). Aging and the societal significance of cohorts. In J. Birren and V. Bengston (Eds.),*Emergent theories of aging*, pp. 405–425. Springer.

Uhlenberg, P. (1992). Population Aging and Social Policy. *Annual Review of Sociology, 18*(1), 449–474. https://doi.org/10.1146/annurev.so.18.080192.002313

Uhlenberg, P. (1996). The burden of aging: A theoretical framework for understanding the shifting balance of caregiving and care receiving as cohorts age. *The Gerontologist, 36*(6), 761-767.

Walker, A. (2013). Intergenerational relations and the provision of welfare. In A. Walker (Ed.) *The new generational contract: Intergenerational relations and the welfare state* (pp. 10-19).University College London Press.

Weller C.E & Newman K (2020) "Increasing Risks, Costs, and Retirement Income Inequality" In J.A. Kelley (ed.) *Annual Review of Gerontology and Geriatrics: inequality in later life*, 40(1). Springer.

Whitbourne, S. K. (1985). The psychological construction of the life span. In J. E. Birren & K. W. Schaie (Eds.), *The handbooks of aging. Handbook of the psychology of aging* (p. 594–618). Van Nostrand Reinhold Co.

Zwick, T. (2012). Training effectiveness–Differences between younger and older employees. *Working and Ageing*, 1752.

Notes

1   In recent years, many self-interested employers have reduced the hours given to "full-time" workers to less than 30 per week, as a way of avoiding the mandated costs of "Obamacare" and other labor regulations. Absent a legislated increase in the current "minimum" wage to a genuine "living wage," however, this has only served to force workers to compensate by taking multiple jobs. On the efficacy of living wage policy in reducing precarity and inequality (see Marshall, 2019; Luce, 2004). The need to transform the current minimum wage policy to a living wage policy is indicated by the fact that the last time the legislated minimum wage could realistically sustain an individual was in the late 1960s (Elwell 2014).

Policy Options to Reduce the Black-White Gap in Retirement Security

Richard W. Johnson, PhD

Urban Institute

rjohnson@urban.org

Acknowledgment: The author gratefully acknowledges financial support from the Alfred P. Sloan Foundation.

Abstract

The racial gap in retirement security is profound. Black people aged 65 and older are four times as likely as their White peers to live in poverty, and on average hold only one-fourth as much household wealth. This deficit has not changed much over the past two decades, but various policy options could help narrow the gap. Shoring up Social Security's finances, boosting Social Security payments to low-income beneficiaries, and expanding Supplemental Security Income would improve financial well-being for many older Black adults. Other policy options, including boosting employment and earnings, facilitating homeownership, and promoting savings could help many younger Black workers build wealth over their lifetime, leaving them more financial secure when they eventually retire.

Keywords: discrimination, income, wealth, inequality, financial status

Opciones de política para reducir la entre negros y blancos en la seguridad de jubilación

Resumen

La brecha racial en la seguridad de la jubilación es profunda. Las personas negras de 65 años o más tienen cuatro veces más probabilidades que sus pares blancos de vivir en la pobreza y, en promedio, poseen solo una cuarta parte de la riqueza familiar. Este déficit no ha cambiado mucho en las últimas dos décadas, pero varias opciones de política podrían ayudar a reducir la brecha. Apoyar las finanzas del Seguro Social, aumentar los pagos del Seguro Social a

doi: 10.18278/jep.1.2.4

los beneficiarios de bajos ingresos y expandir la Seguridad de Ingreso Suplementario mejoraría el bienestar financiero de muchos adultos negros mayores. Otras opciones de políticas, que incluyen aumentar el empleo y los ingresos, facilitar la propiedad de vivienda y promover el ahorro, podrían ayudar a muchos trabajadores negros más jóvenes a acumular riqueza durante su vida, dejándolos más seguros financieramente cuando finalmente se jubilen.

Palabras clave: Brecha racial, jubilación, seguridad social, bienestar financiero

减少黑人-白人退休保障差距的政策选项

摘要

退休保障的种族差距影响深远。65岁及以上的黑人的生活贫困可能性是同龄白人的四倍，并且平均持有的家庭财富仅为后者的四分之一。过去二十年里这种（财富）赤字情况并未发生大的改变，不过，不同政策选项能帮助缩小差距。支持社会保障制度的资金、提高低收入受益者的社会保障金、并扩大社会安全生活补助金（Supplemental Security Income），将改善许多老年黑人的财务状况。其他政策选项，包括提高就业和收入、促进住房自有、提高储蓄，能帮助许多年轻黑人工作者建立财富，当他们最终退休时能拥有更多财务保障。

关键词：种族差距，退休，社会保障制度，财务状况

Financial insecurity at older ages is a growing policy concern. Retirement income largely depends on earnings received at working ages, which determine Social Security benefits, any employer pensions that retirees receive, and the capacity to set aside additional funds for retirement. Although earnings have been growing for women, bolstering their future retirement income, earnings have stagnated over the past few decades for men in the bottom three-fourths of the earnings distribution (Machin, 2016; Rose, 2015), threatening their retirement security. The pillars of the U.S. retirement income system are also under threat. Social Security faces a long-run financial shortfall that could necessitate significant benefit cuts within the next 15 years unless program revenues increase (Board of Trustees, 2020). Traditional employer-provided pensions that provide lifetime annuities to retirees are disappearing, especially in the private sector (Munnell & Sunden, 2004). Spending needs are also increasing at older ages. Retirement savings must last longer as life expectancy increases (Bosley, Morris, & Glen, 2018), more older adults are increasingly entering retirement with significant debt (Butrica & Karamcheva, 2018), and out-of-pocket health care costs are growing at older ages (Hatfield et al., 2018).

Many Black people face special financial challenges in later life. Workers of color generally earn less than their White counterparts, limiting their future Social Security benefits and their ability to save for retirement. Educational deficits reduce wages received by Black workers, but people of color also face systemic racism that limits their employment opportunities and suppresses their earnings (Bertrand & Mullainathan, 2004; Daly, Hobijn, & Pedtke, 2017; Darity & Mason, 1998; Hamilton & Darity, 2012; Penner, 2008; Reid & Rubin, 2005). Black workers also tend to have shorter careers than White workers. Black people's limited employment histories result from health problems, driven at least partly by racism, and caregiving responsibilities that interrupt employment and lead to early retirement (Centers for Disease Control and Prevention, 2013; Feagin & Bennefield, 2014; Fuller-Thomson et al., 2009; Kail, Taylor, & Rogers, 2020; Murphy, Johnson, & Mermin, 2007). Black people are especially likely to serve as primary caregivers for their grandchildren, which can interfere with paid work, raise spending needs, and reduce retirement savings (Chen et al., 2014; Ellis & Simmons, 2014; Minkler & Fuller-Thomson, 2005).

Many people of color also face challenges using their earnings to build wealth. Black workers are less likely than White workers to participate in employer-sponsored retirement plans, an important component of retirement savings, and those who participate contribute less, on average, to their plans (Ariel Investments and Hewitt Associates, 2009; Butrica & Johnson, 2010). Homeownership is an important way to amass wealth, yet rates of homeownership are quite low for people of color (Charles & Hurst, 2002; U.S. Census Bureau, 2020). Moreover, Black homeowners are more likely than White homeowners to hold high-cost mortgages (Bayer, Ferreira, & Ross, 2018), and they are often subject to higher property tax rates (Avenancio-Leon & Howard, 2020). Black people also hold much more student loan debt at ages 25 to 55 than other racial groups (Braga, 2016). The need to service high debt levels, including mortgages and student loans, reduces the availability of resources that can be set aside for retirement (Elliott, Grinstein-Weiss, & Nam, 2013; Rutledge, Sanzenbacher, & Vitagliano, 2016). Black people are less likely than White people to be married (Johnson, Haaga, & Simms, 2011), which allows households to economize on living expenses; to receive inheritances (Hamilton & Darity, 2010), which can help finance home purchases and fund retirement; and to have access to banks, which facilitates saving (Federal Deposit Insurance Corporation, 2018). Consequently, Black families generally hold much less wealth than White families (Dettling et al., 2017; Hou & Sanzenbacher, 2020; Wolf, 2018).

This article documents the financial challenges facing older Black adults and discusses various policy options to improve their financial well-being. We begin by comparing household income and wealth and poverty rates by race and Hispanic origin for adults aged 65 and older. The analysis also reports two-decade trends in income and wealth at older ages, shows how income sources vary by income level, and describes how poverty rates vary by personal characteristics. We then report the share of workers aged 51 to 64 with employer-sponsored retirement plan coverage on their current job.

The tabulations report findings in 2019 inflation-adjusted dollars and use data from the Health and Retirement Study, a nationally representative longitudinal survey of older adults conducted by the Institute for Survey Research at the University of Michigan. When we completed our analysis, the most recent available data were collected in 2016. Because the survey asks respondents about income received in the previous calendar year, our income estimates run through 2015. We adjust for differences in household size by dividing income and wealth estimates for married couples by the square root of 2 (or 1.41). This adjustment factor is commonly used to reflect the higher costs incurred by larger households as well as the savings that result from shared living arrangements (National Research Council, 2005).

The second half of this article discusses policy options that could narrow the racial gap in retirement security. Because many older Black adults rely heavily on Social Security, shoring up the program's finances and boosting payment to low-income beneficiaries would improve their financial well-being at older ages. Expanding Supplemental Security Income (SSI), a federal program that provides cash benefits to needy older adults and people with disabilities, would help many Black retirees. Other policy options, including boosting employment and earnings, facilitating homeownership, and promoting savings, could help younger Black adults build wealth over their lifetime, leaving them better prepared for retirement. Successful implementation of these reforms will require sustained commitment from policymakers and other stakeholders.

The Racial Gap in Economic Well-Being at Older Ages

Older Black adults receive less income than older White adults. They also hold much less wealth, which older adults can draw down to cover living expenses if their incomes fall short. Additionally, Black workers are less likely than White workers to participate in employer-sponsored retirement plans.

Income

Among adults aged 65 and older, median 2015 household income is barely half as much for Black people as White people ($22,100 versus $40,200, measured

86

in 2019 inflation-adjusted dollars) (Table 1). Latinos' median 2015 household income of $17,100 is less than half as much as the median for White people. Within all three groups, about 9 in 10 older adults received Social Security income, but labor earnings, pension income, and asset income were more common among older White people than older people of color. About two-thirds of older White adults received asset income in 2015, for example, compared with less than one-third of Black people and Latinos. Except for other income, which includes means-tested government benefits, the median amount of each income type received was lower for Black people and Latinos than for White people.

The relative importance of different income sources varies with income levels. For all racial groups, Social Security accounted for about four-fifths of 2015 income received by older adults in the bottom third of the income distribution (Table 2). Social Security is less important at higher income levels. Nonetheless, in the middle third of the income distribution it accounted for 80 percent of the income received by older Latinos and 68 percent of the income received by older Black adults (but only 47 percent of the income received by older White adults). In the top third of the income distribution, labor earnings and employer pensions are important sources of income for all groups, and asset income is important for White people.

The racial income gap at older ages has not changed much over the past two decades. At ages 65 to 70, Black median income as a share of White median income increased from 53 percent in 1997 to 61 percent in 2009, but then declined to 49 percent in 2015 in the wake of the 2008 financial crisis and the deep recession that accompanied it (Table 3). For Latinos at ages 65 to 70, median income as a share of White median income fell from 47 percent to 35 percent between 1997 and 2015, with most of the decline occurring after 2009. The racial income gap narrowed slightly between 1997 and 2015 at ages 71 to 76 and ages 77 to 82.

Older Black people are more than four times as likely to be impoverished as older White people. Among adults aged 65 and older, 22 percent of Black people and 28 percent of Latinos had incomes below the federal poverty level (FPL) in 2015, compared with 5 percent of White people (Table 4). The poverty rate was particularly high for older people of color with limited education, adults aged 80 and older, and divorced, widowed, and never married adults. Older women were also more likely than older men to live in poverty, mostly because they were less likely to be married.

Wealth

On average, older Black people and Latinos hold only about one-quarter as much wealth as older White people. In 2016, mean total household wealth, measured in 2019 inflation-adjusted dollars and including the value of housing, other real estate holdings, businesses, automobiles, other modes of transportation, and financial assets minus any outstanding debt, was $159,200 for Black people aged 65 and older, $171,700 for Latinos, and $647,300 for White people (Table 5). Because the wealth distribution is skewed, most older adults hold much less wealth than the average amount. Median household wealth was only $50,600 for older Black adults, $49,600 for older Latinos, and $269,500 for older White adults. One-quarter of older Black people and Latinos had less than $2,500 in wealth.

Most older adults of color hold much of their wealth as home equity. For older Black people, median housing wealth net of outstanding mortgages and other housing debt was $32,000, or 63 percent of their median total wealth. Median net housing wealth equaled 86 percent of median total wealth for older Latinos, but only 39 percent of median total wealth for older White people. Racial wealth disparities are especially pronounced for financial wealth. On average, older Black adults held only 14 percent as much financial wealth as older White adults in 2016, and older Latinos held only 11 percent as much as older Whites. More than one-quarter of older Black people and one-half of older Latinos held no financial assets, and one-half of older Black people had no more than $500 in financial assets. These shortfalls in financial wealth are problematic because most households can easily liquidate much of their financial assets to meet emergencies.

The racial gap in household wealth at older ages has not improved much over the past two decades. Between 1998 and 2016, median total household wealth for Black people as a share of median total wealth for White people fell 4 percentage points at ages 65 to 70, increased 4 percentage points at ages 71 to 76, and fell 7 percentage points at ages 77 to 82 (Table 6). The gap in household wealth between older Latinos and White people narrowed slightly over the past two decades. Latinos' median total household wealth as a share of Whites' median wealth increased 5 percentage points at ages 65 to 70 and ages 71 to 76, and increased 2 percentage points at ages 77 to 82.

Our wealth estimates exclude the expected value of future Social Security benefits. A beneficiary's Social Security wealth can be estimated by summing expected future benefits and discounting those payments that will not be collected for many years because current payments are more valuable than future payments. Social Security is an important asset for most lower-income families, including many Black people, because it replaces a larger share of pre-retirement earnings for beneficiaries with limited lifetime earnings than for those with more earnings. Expanding household wealth measures to include Social Security reduces the racial gap in wealth, although differences remain substantial (Hou & Sanzenbacher, 2020; Wolff, 2018).

Retirement Plan Coverage

Workers of color are less likely than White workers to participate in retirement plans at work, an important vehicle for amassing retirement savings. Among employed workers aged 51 to 64 in 2016, 52 percent of Black people and 37 percent of Latinos were covered by an employer-sponsored retirement plan, compared with 60 percent of White people (Table 7). Coverage rates are higher among full-time workers, but the racial gap is similar. Racial disparities in retirement plan coverage have grown over time. In 1998, coverage rates were similar for Black and White employed workers, whereas the coverage rate for Latino workers lagged only 12 percentage points behind the rate for White workers. For all groups, defined-contribution plans are more common than defined benefit plans, which have become less common over the past two decades.

Policy Options

Various policy options could narrow racial gaps in retirement security. Possibilities include boosting employment and earnings, protecting and improving Social Security, expanding SSI, facilitating home-ownership, and promoting savings.

Improve Employment Outcomes

Narrowing racial gaps in the workplace could substantially improve Black people's financial well-being at older ages, which depends largely on how much people earned earlier in life. More than 50 years after the passage of major Civil Rights legislation intended to reduce racial barriers in employment and education, Blacks continue to earn much less than Whites (Daly, Hobijn, & Pedtke, 2017). Because of these earnings shortfalls, most policies designed to help lower-income workers would disproportionately help Black workers. Options include increasing the minimum wage, expanding apprenticeships, devoting more public funds to workforce development programs, and strengthening labor unions. Labor unions have been declining for decades, but they could be revived by federal policies that facilitate worker efforts to create collective bargaining units, create meaningful penalties for employers who violate labor laws by firing workers who are trying to organize, and overturning state right-to-work laws, which allow employees in unionized workplaces to opt out of union dues.

Other policies and practices would focus more specifically on increasing lifetime earnings for Black workers. Local laws that forbid employers from questioning job applicants about their salary history, which can perpetuate past discrimination and other inequities, have been shown to increase salaries for workers who change jobs, especially women and Black workers (Bessen, Denk, & Meng, 2020). Extending these laws could reduce the racial wage gap. Employers could provide more career mentoring for Black workers and invest more in programs to root out implicit bias in the workplace. To limit unconscious bias in promotion decisions, the U.S. Army no longer shows candidates' photos to officer selection boards (Rempfer, 2020). Eliminating the mass incarceration of Black men would also promote retirement security, because people cannot earn wages, accumulate Social Security credits, or save for retirement when serving time in prison.

Bolster Social Security

Because Social Security accounts for a disproportionate share of the income received by older Black adults, increasing program payments to low-income beneficiaries could substantially improve their financial security. Numerous policymakers, advocates, and policy organizations have advanced proposals to raise Social Security benefits, but they often approach benefit increases differently, affecting the impact on Black beneficiaries. Moreover, Social Security's looming financial problems complicate efforts to increase benefits.

Improve Program Finances

Social Security faces a long-range financing gap driven by reduced fertility and increased life expectancy that has lowered the number of workers supporting each retiree. The program trustees' 2020 intermediate projections indicate that under current rules, Social Security's 75-year shortfall totals 3.21 percent of taxable payroll, and program costs will exceed revenues in 2020 and every subsequent year for the foreseeable future (Board of Trustees, 2020). A large trust fund that built up after 1983, when Congress last addressed Social Security financing, can cover the shortfall for the next decade and a half, but the trustees project that fund reserves will be depleted in 2035. When that happens, the system will be able to cover only about four-fifths of scheduled benefits.

Closing Social Security's long-range financing gap would prevent or at least delay the depletion of the program's trust funds and the need to implement substantial across-the-board benefit cuts. Consequently, steps to bolster Social Security's financial status could prevent or forestall a significant deterioration in the financial security of older adults, including people of color. Policymakers could close the financing gap through some combination of raising revenues and cutting costs. The approach they choose could shape the financial well-being of older Black adults.

Increase the Taxable Maximum. Social Security is financed mainly by payroll taxes.[1] The current payroll tax rate is 6.2 percent, levied on both covered employees and their employers. Self-employed workers pay 12.4 percent of their earnings to the system. However, only earnings in covered employment below the program's contribution and benefit base are subject to taxation each year. That cap, which increases with the growth in the average national wage, was set at $137,700 in 2020.

Many Social Security reform plans, including those proposed by the Bipartisan Policy Center (2016), the National Commission on Fiscal Responsibility and Reform (2010), and many of the 2020 Democratic presidential candidates (Smith, Johnson, & Favreault, 2020), would increase the cap on annual earnings subject to Social Security payroll taxes. Although the program's

---

1   For example, the Social Security 2100 Act (H.R. 860), introduced by Rep. John Larson (D-CT) in 2019, and the Social Security Reform Act of 2016 (H.R. 6489), introduced by then-Rep. Sam Johnson (R-TX), both include minimum benefit provisions.

taxable maximum grows with the average national wage, the share of covered earnings subject to the Social Security payroll tax decreased from 90 percent in 1983 to 83 percent in 2018 because earnings have increased more rapidly for high-wage workers than for moderate- and low-wage workers (Johnson, 2020b). Raising the taxable maximum would move the share of earnings subject to the payroll tax closer to its past level and improve Social Security's financial status.

The financial impact of increasing the taxable maximum would depend on how high the cap is raised, the tax rate applied to higher earnings, and whether workers would receive additional benefit credits for their additional taxes. Some proposals, for example, would eliminate the taxable maximum so that all earnings would be taxed, others would increase the maximum so that the payroll tax covered about 90 percent of earnings, and others would impose additional taxes only on workers with annual earnings above some level, such as $250,000 or $400,000. The Social Security actuaries estimate that removing the taxable maximum in 2021 and later years would eliminate about three-quarters of Social Security's long-range financing gap if the program did not provide benefit credits for those additional taxes and would eliminate only about one-half of the gap if the program provided benefit credits for the additional taxes (Social Security Administration, 2020b). About one-fifth of Social Security's long-range financing shortfall would be eliminated, according to the actuaries, if the tax-

able maximum were increased to cover 90 percent of covered earnings and benefit credits were provided on those contributions. These proposals would not raise taxes on many Black workers because they are much less likely than White workers to earn more than the existing taxable maximum (Favreault & Haaga, 2013).

Other revenue-enhancing proposals for Social Security include raising the payroll tax rate and taxing additional income sources to help finance the program. During the 2020 Democratic presidential primaries, Senator Bernie Sanders (I-VT) and Senator Elizabeth Warren (D-MA) proposed taxing investment income and crediting those revenues to Social Security (Smith, Johnson, & Favreault, 2020). Raising the payroll tax rate would reduce take-home pay for all covered workers, but taxing new income sources might not affect lower- and moderate-income Black workers much if the tax were levied on income sources that mostly go to higher-income workers, such as earnings on investments.

Cut Costs. Another approach to closing Social Security's long-range financing gap is to cut program costs by trimming benefits. One often-proposed option is to trim payments to beneficiaries with high lifetime earnings, which would protect low- and moderate-income Black beneficiaries from benefit cuts.

Another common cost-containment proposal would raise the program's retirement age. In 1983, President Ronald Reagan signed legislation to gradually increase Social Security's full retirement age from 65 to 67. This increase cut benefits by boosting the actuarial reduction for claiming benefits early and reducing the bonus for delaying benefit take-up. Advocates of further raising the full retirement age, which was included in the Social Security Reform Act of 2016 (H.R. 6489), argue that benefits should be cut because most people are living longer. Social Security's actuaries project that increasing the full retirement age to 69 and then increasing it one month every two years thereafter would eliminate slightly more than one-third of the program's long-range financial shortfall (Social Security Administration, 2020c). However, life expectancy has not grown as rapidly for Black people as for White people (Olshansky et al., 2012), so raising the retirement age could disproportionately harm Black people. On the other hand, beneficiaries who first began collecting because of a disability are not subject to actuarial reductions. Those beneficiaries, who are disproportionately Black, would not be harmed by an increase in the retirement age (Mermin & Steuerle, 2006).

Enhance Benefits

Enhancing Social Security benefits could improve retirement security for many people of color. The effectiveness of any such changes would hinge on how policymakers increase benefits.

Create a Meaningful Minimum Benefit. Perhaps the most effective approach

would be to increase Social Security's minimum benefit, which would target benefit increases to those with the smallest benefits (Favreault & Smith, 2020). Social Security currently includes a minimum benefit, designed to support retirees who spent many years working at low wages, but the minimum is too low to help many beneficiaries. At the end of 2019, only 32,100 Social Security beneficiaries received the special minimum, less than one-tenth of 1 percent of all Social Security beneficiaries (Social Security Administration, 2020a). No new Social Security awards have included the special minimum since 1998, except for a few retirees receiving government pensions that reduced their Social Security benefits (Feinstein, 2013). Yet in 2003, 21 percent of Social Security beneficiaries aged 64 to 73 received family Social Security benefits that fell below the FPL, including 43 percent of Black people (Favreault, 2010).

Many prominent Social Security reform proposals would create a meaningful minimum benefit, including proposals from both Democrats and Republicans.[2] The proposed minimum benefit is usually tied to the FPL and years of employment. The Social Security 2100 Act, for example, would set the minimum equal to 125 percent of the FPL for beneficiaries with 30 or more years of covered employment, 100 percent of the FPL for beneficiaries with 26 years of covered employment, and 50 percent of the FPL for beneficia-

---

2   For example, the Social Security 2100 Act (H.R. 860), introduced by Rep. John Larson (D-CT) in 2019, and the Social Security Reform Act of 2016 (H.R. 6489), introduced by then-Rep. Sam Johnson (R-TX), both include minimum benefit provisions.

ries with 18 years of covered employment. One limitation of these proposals, however, is that many older adults with limited Social Security benefits did not have long careers; in 2003, about 9 in 10 beneficiaries aged 64 to 73 receiving benefits below the FPL worked fewer than 30 years in covered employment (Favreault, 2010). Consequently, most beneficiaries who would qualify for the full minimum benefit would fall into the second quintile of the lifetime earnings distribution, not the bottom quintile.

Other Benefit Increases. Other proposals to expand Social Security include across-the-board benefit increases, the introduction of caregiver credits, and increased payments to the survivors of beneficiaries and long-term beneficiaries. The Social Security Expansion Act (S. 478), introduced by Sen. Sanders in 2019, would adjust the Social Security benefit formula to boost payments to all beneficiaries. The benefit formula is progressive; for workers turning 62 in 2020, it replaces 90 percent of their first $960 of average indexed monthly earnings ($11,520 annually), plus 32 percent of the next $4,824 in average monthly earnings, and 15 percent of covered earnings above $5,785 ($69,420 annually), up to the taxable maximum. The Sanders plan would increase the amount of earnings subject to the 90 percent rate.

Another option would supplement the earnings histories that factor into Social Security benefit calculations for workers who take time out of the paid workforce to care for children, dependents with disabilities, or aged family members. The Social Security Caregiver Credit Act of 2019 (S. 2317), introduced by Sen. Chris Murphy (D-CT), would credit workers with one month of earnings equal to one-half of the national average wage for every month that they provided at least 80 hours of care.

Boosting Social Security payments to the survivors of deceased beneficiaries could improve financial security for widows, who are much more likely to live in poverty than married beneficiaries (Johnson, 2020a). Social Security currently offers survivor benefits equal to 100 percent of the deceased spouse's benefit, which would replace the surviving spouse's existing benefit if it generated a larger payment. This survivor benefit is not very valuable when spouses receive similar payments; in those cases, the death of a spouse can reduce household Social Security payments as much as 50 percent. During the 2020 Democratic presidential primary, several candidates, including former Vice President Joe Biden, proposed providing survivors with the option of collecting 75 percent of the total benefit received by the household before the deceased spouse died, as long as that payment did not exceed the benefit received by a two-earner couple with average career earnings (Smith, Johnson, & Favreault, 2020).

Many long-term Social Security beneficiaries receive relatively low payments because their benefits are based on earnings received many years earlier. Social Security's annual cost-of-living adjustment raises payments to offset inflation, but because wages typically grow faster than prices, beneficiaries who began collecting recently generally receive larger benefits than those who began collecting earlier. Moreover, out-of-pocket spending on medical care and home and residential care typically surges after age 80 (Cubanski et al., 2019; Hatfield et al., 2018), exacerbating economic hardship for many long-term beneficiaries. Some Social Security reform proposals would provide a bonus to long-term beneficiaries to improve their financial security. The 2010 plan put forth by the National Commission on Fiscal Responsibility and Reform, for example, would provide a bonus equal to 5 percent of the average benefit to beneficiaries who had collected payments for 20 years; the bonus would phase in, beginning with a 1 percent boost for beneficiaries who had collected for 16 years (Favreault & Karamcheva, 2011).

Boosting payments to widowed beneficiaries would likely help more Black retirees than creating caregiver credits or providing longevity bonuses. Black women are more likely to become widowed than White and Latinx women, even though Black women are less likely to marry (Angel, Jimenez, & Angel, 2007). Caregiver credits tied to average earnings could help people with low earnings, but it could also help higher-income groups who can afford to drop out of the labor force to raise children. Black mothers with young children are more likely to work for pay than White or Latinx mothers (Women's Bureau, U.S. Department of Labor,

2016). Boosting payments to long-term beneficiaries would help White retirees more than Black retirees, because White people tend to live longer (Olshansky et al., 2012). Changing the benefit formula to increase payments to all beneficiaries would not target benefit enhancements to Black people or other groups who may need more help.

Expand Supplemental Security Income

Designed to help people who do not collect Social Security or receive very small payments, SSI provides only limited benefits and enrolls relatively few older adults. The 2020 Federal SSI benefit for an individual is $783 per month, although many states supplement those payments. Recipients without any earnings who do not collect a supplement are left with an income that falls $280 below the FPL. In 2019, only 1.2 million adults aged 65 and older received SSI benefits (Social Security Administration, 2020a), just 2 percent of the U.S. population in that age group. Between 1975 and 2019, as the number of adults aged 65 and older increased by more than 30 million, the number of aged SSI beneficiaries fell by 1.1 million. However, about 8 percent of Black adults aged 65 and older collect SSI, more than twice the rate for White older adults (Favreault, forthcoming).

Expanding SSI could improve Black people's financial security at older ages. Boosting enrollment by simplifying the application procedure and reaching out to potential participants would amplify SSI's impact. Only about one-half to two-thirds of eligible participants enroll in the program (McGarry, 1996; Rupp, Strand, & Davies, 2003). Policymakers could also ease eligibility standards by relaxing SSI's resource test, which permits enrollees to hold no more than $2,000 in countable assets if single and $3,000 if married. Those levels have not increased since 1989, and the resource test excludes only the value of a residence, vehicle, burial plot, household goods, and personal effects. Another option to improve SSI's impact is to increase benefit levels. During her 2020 presidential campaign, Sen. Warren proposed increasing the Federal SSI benefit for individuals to 100 percent of the FPL (Smith, Johnson, & Favreault, 2020).

Facilitate Homeownership

Homeownership helps people build wealth and improve their financial security in old age as they pay off their mortgages. It also often allows people to live in communities with better amenities, including higher-quality schools (Dietz & Haurin, 2003) that can help students obtain good-paying jobs, and it provides families with an important asset that can be passed on to future generations. However, Black people are much less likely than White people to own a home. In the second quarter of 2020, the homeownership rate was 47 percent for Black households, compared with 76 percent for White households (U.S. Census Bureau, 2020). The Black-White homeownership gap narrowed during the 1990s and the first half of the 2000s, as the 1968 Fair Housing Act and subsequent federal legislation outlawed race-based discrimination in access to credit and homeownership, but it increased in the wake of the 2007 financial crisis (Acolin, Lin, & Wachter, 2019). Black households are now only about half as likely as White households to transition from renting to owning a home (Brown & Dey, 2019).

Racial disparities in income, credit scores, and marital status account for much of the Black-White homeownership gap (Acolin, Lin, & Wachter, 2019; Choi et al., 2019). Racial discrimination also appears to play a role, including the legacy of past racist government policies that segregated neighborhoods and restricted Black access to financial credit and homeownership (Rothstein, 2017). The Federal Housing Administration, established in 1934, guaranteed mortgages for homeowners but imposed restrictive covenants in deeds that forbade home sales to Black families. Similarly, the GI Bill, first enacted in 1944 to help veterans returning from World War II buy homes, used the same restrictive practices as the Federal Housing Administration to block homeownership by Black veterans. The impact of these policies continues to linger. By helping to deny the wealth building opportunities that come with homeownership, these policies limited the ability of a generation of Black people to transfer wealth to future generations, making it harder for Black families to buy homes today. The racial homeownership gap today is larger for low-income families, possibly because low-income Black people are less able to count on family help than their White counterparts (Choi et al., 2019). Racial discrimination is not merely a relic of the past. When looking to buy homes, people of color are told about and shown fewer homes by realtors than White people (Turner et al., 2013). Acolin, Desen, and Wachter (2019) find evidence that discrimination may be worsening, as the share of the racial homeownership gap that cannot be explained by differences in financial resources grows.

Policymakers can take several steps to promote Black homeownership (McCargo, Choi, & Golding, 2019). A more equitable housing finance system would help Black people obtain the credit most people need to buy a home. Mortgage credit has become more difficult to obtain after the 2007 global financial crisis (Brown & Dey, 2019), and Black people face higher interest rates than White people (Bartlett et al., 2019). Reforming zoning and land-use regulations could increase the supply of housing, especially at the low end of the market, and make homeownership more affordable, particularly for first-time homebuyers. More outreach to Black renters and counseling on credit building, saving strategies, and the home-buying process could also ease the transition to homeownership.

Promote Savings by Lower-Wage Workers

Changes to the federal income tax code that better reward low- and moderate-income savers could encourage more Black workers to save for retirement. Most retirement savings accumulate in employer-sponsored 401(k)-type accounts that allow workers to deduct their account contributions from their taxable income. These tax deductions are worth more for higher-income savers in high tax brackets than lower-income savers in low tax brackets, and they provide no financial benefit to the estimated 11 percent of working-age adults who do not pay any federal income tax (Fullerton & Rao, 2019). Replacing the tax deduction for saving in tax-qualified retirement accounts with a flat-rate refundable tax credit would strengthen savings incentives for lower-income workers (Butrica et al., 2014).

Another way to help lower-income savers would be to expand the federal Saver's Credit, which currently provides a nonrefundable income tax credit of up to $1,000 ($2,000 if married filing jointly) for low- and moderate-income taxpayers who contribute to a retirement savings account. The credit equals 50 percent, 20 percent, or 10 percent of contributions, depending on taxable income, for those with incomes up to $32,500 (or $65,000 if married filing jointly) in 2020. Making the tax credit fully refundable and raising the income eligibility thresholds would allow more people to benefit from the Saver's Credit.

Saving for retirement is especially challenging for the nearly half of Black workers who lack access to an employer-sponsored retirement plan. Automatic payroll deductions, typically supplemented by employer contributions, allow many workers with 401(k) plans to accumulate significant retirement savings. Several states have recently enacted programs requiring employers that do not provide a retirement plan to automatically enroll their workers in individual retirement accounts (IRAs) and make payroll deductions on their behalf while allowing workers to opt out if they choose (Georgetown University, 2020). Early results from Oregon's plan show that relatively few workers opt out of the plan (Quinby et al., 2019). Expanding these programs to more states or creating a national auto-IRA program could boost retirement saving for many Black workers.

Lack of access to banking services, which limits one's ability to save and obtain credit and raises the cost of financial transactions, also contributes to the racial wealth gap (Altonji & Doraszelski, 2005; Baradaran, 2019). In 2017, 17 percent of Black households were unbanked, meaning that no one in the household had a checking or savings account at an insured institution, compared with only 3 percent of White households (FDIC, 2017.) Another 30 percent of Black households were underbanked, meaning that they had a bank account, but also obtained products or services from an alternative financial services provider. Allowing the postal service to provide simple banking services, such as checking accounts and small loans, could help many Black families save and obtain lower-cost credit (Baradaran, 2019).

Conclusions

Many older Black adults face significant financial challenges. Black people aged 65 and older receive only about half as much income as their White counterparts, and they are more than four times as likely to be impoverished. Average household wealth, including the value of a home, other real property, and financial assets minus outstanding mortgages and other debt, is about four times higher for older White adults than older Black adults. Disparities in financial wealth, which include bank accounts, mutual and money market funds, and stocks and bonds and can generally be easily liquidated in an emergency, are even larger. On average, older White people hold about seven times as much financial wealth as older Black people. The Black-White gap in economic well-being at older ages has not narrowed over the past two decades.

Various policy changes could improve the financial security of older Black adults. Because Social Security accounts for the majority of income received by most Black retirees, shoring up the program's finances may be the most pressing priority. Under current benefit and tax rules, the Social Security trustees project that in 2035 the system's trust funds will run out and Social Security will be able to pay only about four-fifths of scheduled benefits (Board of Trustees, 2020). Those projections were completed before the COVID-19 pandemic plunged the U.S. economy into a deep recession and slashed Social Security revenues, so the program's trust funds may run out sooner. Increasing Social Security revenues, such as by taxing high earnings, could delay or reduce required benefit cuts for Black and other beneficiaries. Social Security benefit enhancements, such as the introduction of a meaningful minimum benefit and increased benefits for the survivors of deceased beneficiaries, and SSI expansions, would also help many Black older adults.

Other policy initiatives could help Black workers accumulate wealth over their lifetimes and improve the financial security of future generations of Black retirees. A more equitable housing finance system that improves access to credit and zoning reforms that increase the supply of affordable housing could enable more Black people to purchase homes and build home equity. Policymakers could promote retirement savings for lower-income workers by expanding the Saver's Credit and incentivizing saving through tax credits instead of tax deductions. Widespread use of auto-IRAs could facilitate retirement savings for workers without access to employer-sponsored retirement accounts. Increasing the minimum wage, expanding apprenticeships, devoting more public funds to workforce development programs, and strength-ening labor unions could increase employment and earnings for many Black workers, allowing more to save for retirement and accumulate additional Social Security credits.

These initiatives could help level the playing field for Black workers and savers, helping them overcome the legacy of racist government policies and ongoing racial discrimination that obstruct wealth building and limit retirement security for many Black people. Some of these policy initiatives would require additional public spending. Expanding Social Security, increasing SSI payments, and investing more in workforce development programs could be expensive and divert resources from other public priorities. Other efforts, such as ensuring that Black people are treated fairly in credit, housing, and labor markets, would not require much funding. Successful implementation of any of these reforms would require sustained commitment from federal, state, and local policymakers and other stakeholders.

References

Acolin, A., Lin, D., & Wachter, S. M. (2019). Endowments and minority home-ownership. *Cityscape, 21*(1), 5–62.

Altonji, J. G., & Doraszelski, U. (2005). The role of permanent income and demographics in black/white differences in wealth. *Journal of Human Resources, 40*(1), 1–30.

Angel, J. L., Jimenez, M. A., & Angel, R. J.. (2007). The economic consequences of widowhood for older minority women. *Gerontologist, 47*(2), 224–34.

Ariel Investments & Hewitt Associates. (2009). *401(k) plans in living color: A study of 401(k) plans across racial and ethnic groups.* https://www.arielinvestments.com/images/stories/PDF/arielhewittstudy_finalweb_7.3.pdf

Avenancio-Leon, C., & Howard, T. (2020). *The assessment gap: Racial inequalities in property taxation.* Hass School of Business, University of California, Berkeley.

Baradaran, M. (2019). *The color of money: black banks and the racial wealth gap.* Harvard University Press.

Bartlett, R., Morse, A., Stanton, R., & Wallace, N.(2019). *Consumer-lending discrimination in the era of fintech.* Hass School of Business, University of California, Berkeley. https://faculty.haas.berkeley.edu/morse/research/papers/discrim.pdf

Bayer, P., Ferreira, F., & Ross, S. L. (2018). What drives racial and ethnic differences in high-cost mortgages? The role of high-risk lenders. *Review of Financial Studies, 31*(1), 175–205.

Bertrand, M., & Mullainathan, S. (2004). Are Emily and Greg more employable than Lakisha and Jamal? A field experiment on labor market discrimination. *American Economic Review, 94*(4), 991–1013.

Bessen, J., Denk, E. & Meng, C. (2020). *Perpetuating inequality: What salary history bans reveal about wages.* Boston University School of Law. http://dx.doi.org/10.2139/ssrn.3628729

Board of Trustees (Board of Trustees, Federal Old-Age and Survivors Insurance and the Federal Disability Insurance Trust Funds). (2020). *The 2020 annual report of the Board of Trustees of the Federal Old-Age and Survivors Insurance and Federal Disability Insurance Trust Funds.* https://www.ssa.gov/OACT/TR/2020/

Bosley, T., Morris, M., & Glenn, K. (2018). *Mortality by career-average earnings level.* Office of the Chief Actuary, Social Security Administration. https://www.ssa.gov/oact/NOTES/pdf_studies/study124.pdf

Braga, B. (2016). *Racial and ethnic differences in family student loan debt.* Urban Institute. https://www.urban.org/research/publication/racial-and-ethnic-differences-family-student-loan-debt

Brown, L. M., & Dey J. (2019, Nov. 7). Role of credit attributes in explaining homeownership gap in the post-crisis period, 2012–2016. 41st Annual Fall Research Conference of the Association for Public Policy Analysis and Management, Denver, CO, United States. https://appam.confex.com/appam/2019/webprogram/Paper32965.html

Butrica, B. A., Harris, B. H., Perun, P., & Steuerle, C. E. (2014). *Flattening tax incentives for retirement saving.* Urban Institute. https://www.urban.org/research/publication/flattening-tax-incentives-retirement-saving

Butrica, B. A., & Johnson, R. W. (2010, June 30). Racial, ethnic, and gender differentials in employer-sponsored pensions. Testimony to the ERISA Advisory Council, U.S. Department of Labor, Washington, DC. https://www.urban.org/research/publication/racial-ethnic-and-gender-differentials-employer-sponsored-pensions

Butrica, B. A., & Karamcheva, N. S. (2018). In debt and approaching retirement: Claim Social Security or work longer? *American Economic Association: Papers and Proceedings, 108,* 401–06.

Georgetown University. (2020). *State initiatives 2020: New programs begin implementation while others consider action.* https://cri.georgetown.edu/states/

Centers for Disease Control and Prevention. (2013). CDC health disparities and inequalities report—United States, 2013. *Morbidity and Mortality Weekly Report, 62*(3), 1-189.

Charles, K. K., & Hurst, E. (2002). The transition to home ownership and the Black-White wealth gap. *Review of Economics and Statistics, 84*(2), 281–97.

Chen, F., Mair, C. A., Bao, L., & Yang, Y. C. (2014). Race/ethnic differentials in the health consequences of caring for grandchildren for grandparents. *Journal of Gerontology B: Social Sciences, 70*(5), 793–803.

Choi, J. H., McCargo, A., Neal, M., Goodman, L., & Young, C. (2019). *Explaining the Black-White homeownership gap: A closer look at disparities across labor markets.* Urban Institute. https://www.urban.org/research/publication/explaining-black-white-homeownership-gap-closer-look-disparities-across-local-markets

Bipartisan Policy Center. (2016). Securing our financial future: Report of the Commission on Retirement Security and Personal Savings. https://bipartisanpolicy.org/wp-content/uploads/2019/03/BPC-Retirement-Security-Report.pdf

Cubanski, J., Koma, W., Damico, A., & Neuman, T. (2019). *How much do Medicare beneficiaries spend out of pocket on health care?* Kaiser Family Foundation. https://www.kff.org/medicare/issue-brief/how-much-do-medicare-beneficiaries-spend-out-of-pocket-on-health-care/

Daly, M. C., Hobijn B., & Pedtke, J. H. (2017). Disappointing facts about the Black-White wage gap. *FRBSF Economic Letter* 2017-26. San Francisco: Federal Bank of San Francisco. https://www.frbsf.org/economic-research/publica

tions/economic-letter/2017/september/disappointing-facts-about-black-white-wage-gap/

Darity Jr., W. A. & Mason, P. L. (1998). Evidence on discrimination in employment: Codes of color, codes of gender. *Journal of Economic Perspectives, 12*(2), 63–90.

Dettling, L. J., Hsu, J. W., Jacobs, L., Moore, K. B. & Thompson, J. P. (2017). *Recent trends in wealth-holding by race and ethnicity: Evidence from the Survey of Consumer Finances.* U.S. Board of Governors of the Federal Reserve System. https://www.federalreserve.gov/econres/notes/feds-notes/recent-trends-in-wealth-holding-by-race-and-ethnicity-evidence-from-the-su vey-of-consumer-finances-20170927.htm

Dietz, R. D., & Haurin, D. R. (2003). The social and private micro-level consequences of homeownership. *Journal of Urban Economics, 54*(3), 401–450.

Elliott, W., Grinstein-Weiss, M., & Nam, I. (2013). *Student debt and declining retirement savings.* Washington University, Center for Social Development.

Ellis, R. R., & Simmons, T. (2014). *Coresident grandparents and their grandchildren: 2012.* U.S. Census Bureau. https://www.census.gov/content/dam/Census/library/publications/2014/demo/p20-576.pdf

Favreault, M. M. (2010). *Workers with low Social Security Benefits: Implications for reform.* Urban Institute. https://www.urban.org/research/publication/workers-low-social-security-benefits-implications-reform

Favreault, M. M. (Forthcoming). *Supplemental Security Income: Continuity and change since 1974.* Urban Institute.

Favreault, M. M., & Haaga, O. G. (2013). *Validating longitudinal earnings in dynamic microsimulation models: The role of outliers.* Urban Institute. https://www.urban.org/research/publication/validating-longitudinal-earnings-dynamic-microsimulation-models-role-outliers

Favreault, M. M., & Karamcheva, N.S. (2011). *How would the President's Fiscal Commission's Social Security Proposals affect future beneficiaries?* Urban Institute. https://www.urban.org/research/publication/how-would-presidents-fiscal-commissions-social-security-proposals-affect-future-benefi ciaries

Favreault, M. M., & Smith, K. E. (2020). *Comparing adequacy adjustments to Social Security.* AARP. https://www.aarp.org/ppi/info-2020/comparing-adequacy-adjustments-to-social-security.html

Feagin, J., & Bennefield, Z. (2014). Systemic racism and U.S. health care. *Social Science and Medicine, 103*, 7–14.

Federal Deposit Insurance Corporation. (2018). *2017 FDIC National Survey of Unbanked and Underbanked Households.* Federal Deposit Insurance Corporation. https://www.fdic.gov/householdsurvey/

Feinstein, C. A. (2013). *Diminishing effect of the special minimum PIA.* Social Security Administration. https://www.ssa.gov/oact/NOTES/pdf_notes/note154.pdf

Fuller-Thomson, E., Nuru-Jeter, A., Minkler, M., & Guralnik, J. M. (2009). Black-White disparities in disability among older Americans: Further untangling the role of race and socioeconomic status. *Journal of Aging and Health, 21*(5), 677–58.

Fullerton, D., & Rao, N. L.(2019). The lifecycle of the 47 percent. *National Tax Journal, 72*(2), 359–96.

Hamilton, D., & Darity Jr., W. A. (2010). Can 'baby bonds' eliminate the racial wealth gap in putative post-racial America? *Review of Black Political Economy, 37*(3-4), 207–16.

Hamilton, D., & Darity Jr., W. A. (2012). Crowded out? The racial composition of American occupations. In J. S. Jackson, C. H. Caldwell, & S. L. Sellers (Eds.), *Researching Black communities: A methodological guide* (pp. 60-78). University of Michigan Press.

Hou, W. & Sanzenbacher, G. T. (2020). *Measuring racial/ethnic retirement wealth inequality.* Center for Retirement Research at Boston College. https://crr.bc.edu/working-papers/measuring-racial-ethnic-retirement-wealth-inequality/

Hatfield, L. A., Favreault, M. M., McGuire, T. G., & Chernew, M. E. (2018). Modeling health care spending growth of older adults. *Health Services Research, 53*(1), 138–55.

Johnson, R. W. (2020a). Financial challenges at older ages and the implications for housing options. *Generations,* Summer 2020. https://generations.asaging.org/class-race-housing-challenges-fiscal-challenges

Johnson, R. W. (2020b). *How does earnings inequality affect Social Security financing?* AARP. https://www.aarp.org/ppi/info-2020/how-does-earnings-inequality-affect-social-security-financing.html

Johnson, R. W., Haaga, O., & Simms, M. (2011). *50+ African American workers: A status report, implications, and recommendations.* AARP. https://assets.aarp.org/rgcenter/econ/aa-workers-11.pdf

Kail, B. L., Taylor, M. G., & Rogers, N. (2020). Double disadvantage in the process of disablement: Race as a moderator in the association between chronic conditions and functional limitations. *Journal of Gerontology: Social Sciences, 75*(2), 448–58.

Machin, S. (2016). Rising wage inequality, real wage stagnation, and unions. *Research in Labor Economics, 43*, 329–54.

McCargo, A., Choi, J. H., & Golding, E. 2019. *Building black homeownership bridges: A five-point framework for reducing the racial homeownership gap.* Urban. Institute. https://www.urban.org/research/publication/building-black-homeownership-bridges

McGarry, K. (1996). Factors determining participation of the elderly in Supplemental Security Income. *Journal of Human Resources, 31*(2), 331–58.

Mermin, G. B. T., & Steuerle, C. E. (2006). *Would raising the Social Security retirement age harm low-income groups?* Urban Institute. https://www.urban.org/research/publication/would-raising-social-security-retirement-age-harm-low-income-groups

Minkler, M., & Fuller-Thomson, E. (2005). African American grandparents raising grandchildren: A national study using the Census 2000 American Community Survey. *Journals of Gerontology B: Psychological Sciences and Social Sciences, 60*(2), S82–92.

Munnell, A. H., & Sunden, A. (2004). *Coming up short: The challenge of 401(k) plans.* Brookings Institution Press.

Murphy, D., Johnson, R. W., & Mermin, G. B. T. **(2007).** *Racial differences in baby boomers' retirement expectations.* Urban Institute. https://www.urban.org/research/publication/racial-differences-baby-boomers-retirement-expectations

National Commission on Fiscal Responsibility and Reform. (2010). *The moment of truth: Report of the National Commission on Fiscal Responsibility and Reform.*

National Research Council. (2005). *Measuring poverty: A new approach.* National Academies Press.

Olshansky, S. J., Antonucci, T., Berkman, L., Binstock, R. H., Boersch-Supan, A., Cacioppo, J. T., Carnes, B. A., et al. (2012). Differences in life expectancy due to race and educational differences are widening, and many may not catch up. *Health Affairs, 31*(8), 1803–13.

Penner, A. M. (2008). Race and gender differences in wages: The role of occupational sorting at the point of hire. *Sociological Quarterly, 49*(3), 597–614.

Quinby, L. D., Munnell, A. H., Hou, W., Belbase, A., & Sanzenbacher, G. T. (2019). *Participation and pre-retirement withdrawals in Oregon's auto-IRA*. Center for Retirement Research at Boston College. https://crr.bc.edu/working-pa pers/participation-and-pre-retirement-withdrawals-in-oregons-auto-ira/

Reid, L. W., & Rubin, B. A. (2005). Integrating economic dualism and labor market segmentation: The effects of race, gender, and structural location on earn-ings, 1974–2000. *Sociological Quarterly, 44*(3), 405–432.

Rempfer, K. (2020, June 25). Army ditches officer promotion photos as part of an effort to eliminate unconscious bias. *Army Times.* https://www.armytimes. com/news/your-army/2020/06/25/army-ditches-promotion-photos-as-part-of-an-effort-to-eliminate-unconcious-bias/

Rose, S. (2015). *Beyond the wage stagnation story.* Urban Institute. https:// www.urban.org/sites/default/files/publication/65351/2000331-Be yond-the-Wage-Stagnation-Story.pdf

Rothstein, R. (2017). *The color of law: A forgotten history of how our government segregated America.* Liveright Publishing.

Rupp, K., Strand, A., & Davies, P. S. (2003). Poverty among elderly women: As-sessing SSI options to strengthen Social Security reform. *The Journals of Gerontology: Series B, 58*(6), S359–68.

Rutledge, M. S., Sanzenbacher, G. T., & Vitagliano, F. M. (2016). *How does stu-dent debt affect early career retirement saving?* Center for Retirement Re-search at Boston College. https://crr.bc.edu/wp-content/uploads/2016/09/ wp_2016-9_rev.pdf

Smith, K. E., Johnson, R. W., & Favreault, M. M. (2020). *Five Democratic ap-proaches to Social Security reform: Estimated impact of plans from the 2020 presidential campaign.* Urban Institute. https://www.urban.org/research/ publication/five-democratic-approaches-social-security-reform-estimat-ed-impact-plans-2020-presidential-campaign

Social Security Administration. (2020a). *Annual statistical supplement to the Social Security Bulletin, 2020.* https://www.ssa.gov/policy/docs/statcomps/sup plement/

Social Security Administration. (2020b). *Provisions affecting payroll taxes.* Social Security Administration. https://www.ssa.gov/oact/solvency/provisions/ payrolltax.html

Social Security Administration. (2020c). *Provisions affecting retirement age.* Social Security Administration. https://www.ssa.gov/oact/solvency/provisions/ retireage.html#C1

Turner, M. A., Santos, R., Levy, D. K., Wissoker, D., Aranda, C., & Pitingolo, R. (2013). *Housing discrimination against racial and ethnic minorities 2012.* Office of Policy Development and Research, U.S. Department of Housing and Urban Development. https://www.huduser.gov/portal/Publications/pdf/HUD-514_HDS2012.pdf

U.S. Census Bureau. (2020). Quarterly residential vacancies and homeownership, second quarter 2020. https://www.census.gov/housing/hvs/files/currenth vspress.pdf

Wolff, E. N. (2018). *The decline of African-American and Hispanic wealth since the Great Recession.* National Bureau of Economic Research. https://www.nber.org/papers/w25198

Women's Bureau, U.S. Department of Labor. (2016). *Labor force participation rates.* https://www.dol.gov/agencies/wb/data/latest-annual-data/labor-force-participation-rates

Table 1. Adjusted Household Income by Source, Race, and Hispanic Origin, 2015

Adults aged 65 and older

	Black	**Latinx**	**White**
Median adjusted household income ($)	22,100*	17,100*	40,200
Percentage with income			
Social Security	90*	89*	93
Labor earnings	24*	19*	28
Pension income	36*	27*	54
Asset income	31*	23*	66
Other income	41	37	38
Median amount among those receiving income ($)			
Social Security	13,800*	13,400*	18,500
Labor earnings	24,400	22,100*	31,500
Pension income	12,900	10,800*	13,800
Asset income	700*	2,600	2,400
Other income	4,000*	2,300*	1,200

Source: Author's calculations from the Health and Retirement Study.

Notes: Financial amounts are reported in 2019 inflation-adjusted dollars. The analysis divides reported household income by the square root of 2 for married adults, to reflect the greater spending needs of couples relative to single adults. Asset income includes business or farm income, self-employment earnings, rent, dividend and interest income, and income from trust funds and royalties. Pension income includes income from employer-sponsored pensions and annuities. Other income includes income from alimony, unemployment insurance, workers' compensation, other government benefits, and lump sums from insurance, pensions, and inheritances.

* indicates that the estimate differs significantly from the corresponding estimate for White people ($p < .05$)

Table 2. Composition of Adjusted Household Income by Income Tercile, Race, and Hispanic Origin, 2015 (%)

Adults aged 65 and older

	Black	Latinx	White
Bottom third			
Social Security	79	82	80
Labor earnings	2	2	2
Pension income	3	3	9
Asset income	1	2	4
Other income	15	12	4
Middle third			
Social Security	68	80	47
Labor earnings	6	4	11
Pension income	13	5	26
Asset income	4	1	10
Other income	10	9	6
Top third			
Social Security	23	25	13
Labor earnings	33	32	28
Pension income	26	17	15
Asset income	9	19	31
Other income	9	8	13

Source: Author's calculations from the Health and Retirement Study.

Notes: The analysis divides reported household income by the square root of 2 for married adults, to reflect the greater spending needs of couples relative to single adults. Asset income includes business or farm income, self-employment earnings, rent, dividend and interest income, and income from trust funds and royalties. Pension income includes income from employer-sponsored pensions and annuities. Other income includes income from alimony, unemployment insurance, workers' compensation, other government benefits, and lump sums from insurance, pensions, and inheritances. Income terciles are estimated separately for each racial group.

Table 3. Trends in Median Adjusted Total Household Income by Age, Race, and Hispanic Origin, 1997-2015 ($)

	Dollar Amount			As a Percentage of White Income	
	Black	Latinx	White	Black	Latinx
Aged 65-70					
1997	21,100*	18,900*	40,000	53	47
2003	25,000*	20,300*	43,500	57	47
2009	27,000*	19,600*	44,000	61	45
2015	27,600*	19,800*	55,900	49	35
Aged 71-76					
1997	18,900*	15,400*	32,800	58	47
2003	19,200*	16,700*	34,600	55	48
2009	21,500*	16,000*	36,400	59	44
2015	24,300*	21,400*	39,600	61	54
Aged 77-82					
1997	18,900*	15,400*	32,800	58	47
2003	19,200*	16,700*	34,600	55	48
2009	21,500*	16,000*	36,400	59	44
2015	24,300*	21,400*	39,600	61	54

Source: Author's calculations from the Health and Retirement Study.

Notes: Financial amounts are reported in 2019 inflation-adjusted dollars. The analysis divides reported household income by the square root of 2 for married adults, to reflect the greater spending needs of couples relative to single adults.

* indicates that the estimate differs significantly from the corresponding estimate for White people ($p < .05$)

Table 4. Poverty Rates by Personal Characteristics, Race, and Hispanic Origin, 2015

Adults aged 65 and older

	Black	Latinx	White
All	22*	28*	5
Education			
Did not complete high school	33*	38*	13
High school graduate	19*	15*	5
College graduate	13*	16*	3
Age			
65-69	19*	31*	4
70-74	17*	19*	3
75-79	23*	24*	5
80 and older	32*	37*	8
Gender			
Male	18*	21*	3
Female	25*	32*	6
Marital status and gender			
Married	6*	19*	2
Not married	32*	39*	10
Men	34*	26*	8
Women	31*	44*	11

Source: Author's calculations from the Health and Retirement Study.

Notes: Table shows the share of adults aged 65 and older with incomes below 100 percent of the federal poverty line.

* indicates that the estimate differs significantly from the corresponding estimate for White people ($p < .05$)

Table 5. Adjusted Household Wealth by Type, Race, and Hispanic Origin, 2016

Adults aged 65 and older

	Dollar amount			As a Percentage of White Adults	
	Black	**Latinx**	**White**	**Black**	**Latinx**
Total household wealth					
Mean	159,200*	171,700*	647,300	25	27
25th percentile	2,100*	2,400*	86,600	2	3
50th percentile (median)	50,600*	49,600*	269,500	19	18
75th percentile	154,400*	177,100*	675,400	23	26
Net housing wealth					
Mean	75,900*	94,500*	158,600	48	60
25th percentile	0*	0*	26,600	0	0
50th percentile (median)	32,000*	42,600*	105,500	30	40
75th percentile	95,900*	117,200*	207,700	46	56
Financial wealth					
Mean	44,900*	37,000*	323,400	14	11
25th percentile	0*	0*	5,300	0	0
50th percentile (median)	500*	0*	76,800	1	0
75th percentile	8,800*	7,500*	323,900	3	2

Source: Author's calculations from the Health and Retirement Study.

Notes: Table reports wealth in 2019 inflation-adjusted dollars and divides household wealth by the square root of 2 for married adults, to reflect the greater spending needs of couples relative to single adults. Total household wealth includes the value of housing, other real estate holdings, businesses, automobiles and other modes of transportation, and financial assets, minus any outstanding debt. Net housing wealth includes the value of the primary residence minus any outstanding mortgages. Financial wealth includes the value of stocks, mutual funds, money market funds, checking and savings accounts, certificates of deposit, bonds, individual retirement accounts, Keogh plans, annuities, and other financial assets.

* indicates that the estimate differs significantly from the corresponding estimate for White people ($p < .05$)

Table 6. Trends in Median Adjusted Total Household Wealth by Age, Race, and Hispanic Origin, 1998-2016

	Dollar Amount			As a Percentage of White Wealth	
	Black	Latinx	White	Black	Latinx
Aged 65-70					
1998	49,900*	34,200*	240,800	21	14
2004	56,500*	60,800*	290,600	19	21
2010	69,800*	42,300*	284,000	25	15
2016	46,800*	52,700*	283,300	17	19
Aged 71-76					
1998	44,400*	45,500*	225,700	20	20
2004	54,100*	46,700*	281,400	19	17
2010	59,500*	51,400*	264,200	23	19
2016	67,100*	70,800*	281,000	24	25
Aged 77-82					
1998	46,300*	31,400*	199,800	23	16
2004	35,300*	76,600*	268,000	13	29
2010	62,700*	7,000*	274,600	23	3
2016	45,200*	49,600*	278,000	16	18

Source: Author's calculations from the Health and Retirement Study.

Notes Table reports wealth in 2019 inflation-adjusted dollars and divides household wealth by the square root of 2 for married adults, to reflect the greater spending needs of couples relative to single adults. Total household wealth includes the value of housing, other real estate holdings, businesses, automobiles and other modes of transportation, and financial assets, minus any outstanding debt.

* indicates that the estimate differs significantly from the corresponding estimate for White people (*p* < .05)

Table 7. Retirement Plan Coverage on the Current Job, by Type, Race, and Hispanic Origin, 1998 and 2016 (%)

Workers aged 51 to 64

	Black	Latinx	White
All employed workers			
Any coverage			
1998	56	46*	58
2016	52*	37*	60
Defined-benefit plans			
1998	36	23*	33
2016	19*	16*	27
Defined-contribution plans			
1998	26*	27*	37
2016	38*	21*	43
Full-time workers			
Any coverage			
1998	64	54*	67
2016	61*	44*	69
Defined-benefit plans			
1998	41	28*	40
2016	23*	20*	31
Defined-contribution plans			
1998	30*	32*	44
2016	45*	25*	50

Source: Author's calculations from the Health and Retirement Study.

Notes: The analysis defines full-time work as 35 or more hours per week.

* indicates that the estimate differs significantly from the corresponding estimate for White people ($p < .05$)

Health Advocacy and Health Communication for Elderly Health Care Consumers: Rationale, Demand, and Policy Implications

Gary L. Kreps, PhD
George Mason University, Department of Communication
gkreps@gmu.edu

ABSTRACT

Health advocacy is an important set of communication activities to promote the best health outcomes for individuals confronting health threats, especially for elderly health care consumers, who utilize high levels of health care services for both chronic and acute health problems. However, many elderly health care consumers do not receive adequate advocacy support and have difficulty shaping health care policies and practices due to problems with ageism and power imbalances within health care systems, which accord far more authority to health care providers and administrators than to consumers in the delivery of care. This limits elders' participation and influence in health care, despite research showing that active consumer involvement usually improves health outcomes. Strategic health advocacy can rebalance power within health care, developing and refining health policies and practices. The best advocacy actively represents the voices, concerns, and needs of consumers within health care systems to help make programs responsive to consumer needs. Health advocates must effectively communicate patients' perspectives and needs to key audiences using strategic message strategies and channels to influence health policies and practices. Yet effective advocacy does not happen naturally and needs to be nurtured by relevant programs and policies to represent consumer needs for enhancing health outcomes for elderly health care consumers.

Keywords: Supporting Patient Needs, Social Support, Health Care Bureaucracy, Caregiving, Empowerment

doi: 10.18278/jep.1.2.5

Defensa de la salud y comunicación de salud para consumidores de atención médica de ancianos: Fundamentos, demanda e implicaciones de políticas

Resumen

La promoción de la salud es un conjunto importante de actividades de comunicación para promover los mejores resultados de salud para las personas que enfrentan amenazas para la salud, especialmente para los consumidores de atención médica de edad avanzada, que utilizan altos niveles de servicios de atención médica para problemas de salud tanto crónicos como agudos. Sin embargo, muchos consumidores de atención médica de edad avanzada no reciben el apoyo de defensa adecuado y tienen dificultades para dar forma a las políticas y prácticas de atención médica debido a problemas de discriminación por edad y desequilibrios de poder dentro de los sistemas de atención médica, que otorgan mucha más autoridad a los proveedores y administradores de atención médica que a los consumidores en la prestación de cuidados. Esto limita la participación e influencia de los ancianos en la atención médica, a pesar de que las investigaciones muestran que la participación activa de los consumidores generalmente mejora los resultados de salud. La promoción de la salud estratégica puede reequilibrar el poder dentro de la atención de la salud, desarrollando y perfeccionando las políticas y prácticas de salud. La mejor promoción representa activamente las voces, preocupaciones y necesidades de los consumidores dentro de los sistemas de atención médica para ayudar a que los programas respondan a las necesidades de los consumidores. Los defensores de la salud deben comunicar eficazmente las perspectivas y necesidades de los pacientes a las audiencias clave utilizando estrategias y canales de mensajes estratégicos para influir en las políticas y prácticas de salud. Sin embargo, la promoción efectiva no ocurre de forma natural y debe nutrirse de programas y políticas relevantes para representar las necesidades de los consumidores para mejorar los resultados de salud de los consumidores de atención médica de edad avanzada.

Palabras clave: defensa de la salud, grupos y organizaciones de defensa, toma de decisiones informada, liderazgo, comunicación sobre la salud, defensa de los medios

针对老年医疗消费者的卫生倡导和卫生传播：原理、需求及政策意义

摘要

卫生倡导是一系列重要的传播活动，用于为面对健康威胁的个体，尤其是老年医疗消费者（高度使用医疗服务治疗慢性和急性健康问题）推动最佳卫生结果。不过，许多老年医疗消费者没有获得足够的倡导支持，并且由于医疗系统内部的年龄歧视和权力不平衡而无法顺利影响医疗政策及实践，这种医疗系统在提供护理的过程中将更多权力交给医疗供应商和管理者，而不是消费者。此举限制了老年人在医疗中的参与和影响，尽管研究表明，积极的消费者参与通常能改善卫生结果。战略性卫生倡导能重新平衡医疗中的权力分配，发展并改进卫生政策及实践。最佳倡导能积极代表医疗系统中消费者的声音、顾虑和需求，以期帮助创造能照顾消费者需求的计划。卫生倡导者必须将病人的视角和需求有效传播给关键受众，使用战略性信息策略和渠道来影响卫生政策及实践。不过，有效的倡导不会自然发生，需要通过相关计划和政策加以培养，以期代表消费者需求，为老年医疗消费者改善卫生结果。

关键词：卫生倡导，倡导团体和组织，知情决策，领导力，卫生传播，媒体倡导

Introduction: Health Advocacy and the Health Care System

Health advocacy is a critically important set of communication activities that provide needed information and support for health care consumers to help them negotiate the complexities of health care systems to achieve their best health outcomes from serious health threats (Kreps, 2013; Kreps & Kim, 2013). The modern health care system, which is composed of myriad health care delivery, financ-ing, training, staffing, supply, and regulatory organizations, can be a complex, bureaucratic, and frightening landscape for patients to navigate, especially when patients are incapacitated with serious health problems that lead to pain, fatigue, nausea, imbalance, incontinence, and/or confusion that make it difficult for them to speak-up and participate actively in directing their own care. In these challenging circumstances, health advocates can provide tremendous support for elderly patients by standing up for and representing patents, who are often incapacitated by their health conditions, to help them accomplish their health care needs and wishes. A growing body of compelling empirical evidence illustrates that effective health advocacy services significantly enhance health outcomes for vulnerable patients (Dillardet al., 2018; Dohan & Shrag, 2005; Greenfield, Kaplan, & Ware, 1985; Kahanaet al., 2010; Kreps, 2003; Kreps & Chapelsky Massimilla, 2002; Kreps & O'Hair, 1995; Kreps & Sivaram, 2010; Mattson & Lam, 2015; Natale-Pereira et al.2011; Sklar, 2016; Thomas, 2019). Yet there still are limited health advocacy resources for many elderly patients, as well as insufficient relevant and effective policies and programs to promote, support, and sustain health advocacy services for consumers within the modern health care system (Conrad et al.,2019; Godinho, Murthy, & Ciraj, 2017; Sklar, 2016).

Health advocacy services are especially relevant for elderly health care consumers who often need support in navigating the increasingly complex and bureaucratic modern health care system (Kreps, 1996; 2012; 2013). Elders have a major stake in the quality of health care delivery programs since they utilize high levels of health care services for a wide variety of challenging chronic and acute health problems (Cheng et al., 2020). Sadly, elderly patients often are not accorded high levels of status and respect within health care systems due to problems with ageism and paternalism (Banerjee, D'Cruz, & Rao, 2020; Hooker et al.,2019; Kreps, 1986; 1990; Wyman, Shiovitz-Ezra, & Bengel, 2018). Moreover, elderly individuals confront many challenging health risks, often have low resistance to infectious diseases, and are also often highly susceptible to poor health outcomes (Beardet al., 2016; Cheng et al., 2020). For example, during the COVID-19 pandemic, elderly individuals were found to be at extremely high risk for both contagion and serious negative health outcomes from the coronavirus, including high levels of morbidity and mortality (Ayalon et al.,2020; Banerjee, D'Cruz, & Rao, 2020; Colendaet al., 2020; Morgan & Reid, 2020). Elderly COVID-19 patients often depended heavily on the help of health advocates and health advocacy groups to access needed care and support to confront the deadly disease (Banerjee, D'Cruz, & Rao, 2020; Blyskal, 2020; D'Cruz & Banerjee, 2020; Flatharta & Mulkerrin, 2020). This article examines the powerful role that health advocacy can perform as a critically important form of communication to enhance health outcomes for elderly health care consumers and explores how relevant programs and policies can support health advocacy services.

The Need for Health Advocacy in Modern Health Care

The modern health care system can be confusing, intimidating, and frightening for many consumers (patients and their significant others), but especially for many elderly patients, and there are often limited robust communication mechanisms for providing clear and easy access to relevant information and support to consumers for dealing with complex health problems (Kreps, 2012; 1996; 1990; 1986; Sundler et al.,2020). Communication from health care providers to consumers is often highly technical and specialized, so only those patients with especially high levels of health literacy can comprehend available messages that contain health information relevant to their care (Kreps, 2018; 1988). Elderly patients, in particular, often need help from individuals with high levels of health literacy who can explain to them critically important, but often very complex information about disease prevention, diagnosis, and treatment so these patients can make informed health decisions (Kreps, 1986; 1988; 1990; 2018; Kreps, Neuhauser, Sparks, & Labelle, 2020). Health advocates are adept at helping to perform this important information sharing function for health care consumers (Darien, 2016; Harris, Bayer, & Tadd, 2002).

Elderly health care consumers, in particular, also often face significant personal challenges in participating in directing their own care, helping to shape health care policies and practices related to their care (Adelman, Greene, & Silva, 2017; Stewart, Meredith, Brown, & Galajda, 2000). These health communication barriers are grounded in serious longstanding communication and power imbalances within the health care system that accord far more influence over health care decision-making to health care providers and administrators than to consumers (Banerjee, D'Cruz, & Rao, 2020; Edley & Battaglia, 2016; Leontiou, 2020). There are additional serious communication barriers

that limit elderly patients' active participation in and direction of their own care that are often related to problems with ageist and stereotypic perceptions of the elderly, such as limited opportunities to express their wishes and have their voices heard concerning their health care concerns and preferences, difficulties in establishing truly collaborative patient-provider relationships, challenges to understanding complex health information due to health literacy issues, and problems with paternalism within the health care system that lead to serious power imbalances (Adelman, Greene, & Silva, 2017; Edley & Battaglia, 2016; Leontiou, 2020; Colendaet al., 2020; Wyman, Shiovitz-Ezra, & Bengel, 2018).

Traditional power imbalances limit consumer participation and influence within the modern health care system despite a large body of literature that has shown that increases in active patient participation in health care and health promotion efforts can significantly improve important health outcomes (Greenfield, Kaplan, & Ware, 1985; Kreps, 1988; 2012a; 2017; Kreps, & Chapelsky Massimilla, 2002; Kreps & O'Hair, 1995; Kreps & Sivaram, 2008; Stewart et al.,2000; Street et al.,2009). Elderly patient participation in health care decision-making is often constrained by the limited expectations health care providers have about elders' abilities to participate meaningfully in health care deliberations, problems providers may have in communicating effectively with their elderly patients, and physical challenges elderly patients may have that are related to their health conditions (Banerjee, D'Cruz, & Rao, 2020; Colenda et al., 2020; Schroyen et al.,2018). Health advocacy has the potential to help ameliorate many of the challenges that elderly health care consumers regularly confront within health care systems (Kahanaet al., 2010; Kahana, & Langendoerfer, 2018; Kreps, 2013).

The Process of Health Advocacy

Health advocacy involves the use of strategic communication practices that typically occur on two major levels of the health care system, the individual and the organizational levels (Kreps, 2013). On the individual level, health advocates communicate directly with specific patients (and their caregivers) to promote quality of care and informed decision-making for these consumers (Kreps, 2013). On the organizational level, advocacy groups and organizations engage in directed communication activities to represent the health needs of consumers who confront similar health challenges. Both the individual and organizational levels of advocacy depend on effective and strategic health communication to help promote the best health outcomes for elderly patients (Kreps, 2013; Mattson, & Lam, 2015).

The Individual Level of Health Advocacy

On the individual level of health advocacy, Personal Health Advocates (PHAs) work closely with patients and their supporters to provide relevant health information and support in the pursuit of needed care. PHAs are sometimes trained health navigators, health assistants, and health care providers, but most often health advocacy services are provided informally by untrained, but often highly dedicated, familial caregivers and friends (Petronio et al., 2004). Kahana and Kahana (2003) refers to these informal advocates as health significant others (HSOs), who often accompany patients to health care appointments and represent elderly patients, when needed, with relevant health care providers and administrators. Informal HSOs typically serve as personal advocates for elderly loved ones when they face serious health challenges and have difficulty representing their own health needs, perhaps due to reduced physical or mental capacity related to their health conditions or due to limited health decision-making authority, such as the reduced decision-making authority that young children and incapacitated elderly patients often experience (Berger, 2020; Gray, Nolan, Clayman, & Wenzel, 2019; Kahana & Kahana, 2003; Petronio et al., 2004). Due to these challenges many patients can benefit from effective personal health advocacy, and there is tremendous potential for both informal and formal health advocates to assist patients who are seeking health care services. Informal PHAs often do not only help patients in clinical settings, but also help patients at home adopt and maintain healthy behaviors to reduce significant health risks through reminders, reinforcement, education, support, and encouragement. The best informal PHAs are likely to be those who have high levels of health literacy and are familiar with the workings of the modern health care system (Bell, Whitney, & Young, 2019; Kinsella-Meier, 2019; Kreps, 2013; Moss, 2017).

Individual level health advocacy is also often delivered by formally trained health care professionals, including health navigators, consumer advocates, patient educators, home health nurses, personal trainers, social workers, chaplains, and even physicians who work closely with their patients to help promote their best possible health outcomes (Kahana et al.,2018; Luft, 2017; Schwartz, 2002; Soklaridis et al., 2018; Teague et al., 2019). Kahana, Yu, Kahana, and Langendoerfer (2018) found that elderly patients generally prefer having their personal physicians serve as PHAs for them since they trust their physicians to look out for their interests and are confident that their physicians have the requisite knowledge to effectively navigate the complex health care situations. Research has demonstrated that formal health advocates can dramatically enhance health consumer satisfaction, understanding, quality of care, and improve important health outcomes (Dohan & Schragg, 2005; Natale-Pereira et al., 2011). Yet the need for health advocacy services outruns the availability of such services, resulting in a tremendous need to develop relevant programs and policies to support formal delivery of health advocacy in health care systems to make sure that the best advocacy services are available and provided to elderly patients who need support (Dillard et al., 2018; Kreps & Kim, 2013; Thomas, 2019).

Individual level health advocacy, delivered both informally and formally, can provide valuable support for elderly health care consumers to help these consumers receive relevant health information, advice, and the best care to promote their health and well-being. PHAs depend on their strategic communication skills to gather relevant information concerning elderly consumer's health concerns, interpret health care recommendations and advice, share this information clearly and compellingly with consumers, and to serve as a liaison between consumers, health care providers, family members, and health care system administrators (Kreps, 2013; Mattson, & Lam, 2015). PHAs often serve a multitude of specific functions for elderly patients, including making an array of arrangements for patients within health care delivery systems, helping to schedule patient health care services and appointments, coordinating care from different specialists (such as, therapists, surgeons, nutritionists, pharmacists, and many others), accompanying patients to appointments, arranging patient transportation to health care settings, negotiating health care billing issues, picking up and delivering medications and health care supplies for patients, providing patients with relevant health information in ways patients can understand to help patients make informed health decisions, filling out needed forms, explaining patients' perspectives to health care providers and administrators, answering patients' questions about health advice provided to them by health care providers, and searching for relevant health information for patients (Kreps, 2013; Mattson & Lam, 2015).

Organizational Level Health Advocacy

The organizational level of health advocacy involves Health Advocacy Groups and Organizations (HAGOs) that raise money to fund research, education, treatment, and support services related to health care and health promotion for health care consumers (Kreps & Kim, 2013; Kreps et al., 2012; 2013). HGOs often lobby government agencies and health care systems to help establish relevant health care delivery regulations and programs to support the health needs of patients who these organizations represent. HAGOs often establish important patient education and support programs and resources for patients and for patient caregivers. They also encourage (and sometimes fund) needed health research to expand knowledge, prevention, and treatment for the health care issues their members face. Formal advocacy organizations also can help to facilitate refinements in health care delivery system programs, practices, and policies. Some of the larger and most well-established health advocacy organizations have become familiar names to the public, such as the American Cancer Society, the Susan Komen Foundation, the Alzheimer's Association, the American Heart Association, the National Kidney Foundation, and the National Alliance on Mental Illness. These HAGOs often serve the needs of elderly health care consumers (both patients and their health significant others), and these ad-

vocacy organizations have become particularly important for helping elderly patients navigate the complex health care challenges they have faced recently during the COVID-19 pandemic (Banerjee, D'Cruz, & Rao, 2020; D'Cruz & Banerjee, 2020).

There are also narrowly focused HAGOs that support the needs of patients and families confronting specific health care concerns, such as the Alzheimer's Association, the Pancreatic Cancer Action Network, and the Susan G. Komen Breast Cancer Foundation. Both the broader and more narrowly focused HAGOs are complex organizational enterprises that depend on strategic communication activities to support health care consumer needs, such as working cooperatively with media representatives to raise awareness about key health issues of importance to their members, advancing the growth of health care knowledge and disseminating new information about the diseases they represent to key audiences, engaging in the design and implementation of complex fundraising and health promotion campaigns, and working collaboratively with key representatives of health care delivery systems and health research organizations (Kreps, 2013; Mattson & Lam, 2015; Wallack et al.,1999).

There is a long history of cancer-related health advocacy activities in the U.S. that have powerfully influenced relevant health care research, as well as the development of important health policies and practices that are relevant to addressing the health needs of elderly consumers (Kim, 2007). Cancer is largely a disease of aging, so many cancer advocacy organizations very actively serve the needs of elderly cancer patients and their caregivers (Anisimov, 2020; Levit, Singh, & Klepin, 2020; Lund, 2019). For example, the American Cancer Society (ACS), which was founded in 1913 as the American Society for the Control of Cancer by a group of prominent physicians and business leaders, has developed many influential programs to enhance the quality of cancer care and provide support to cancer patients. Prominent individuals have also had major influences on consumer advocacy by establishing influential health advocacy organizations. For example, Mary Woodward Lasker, who founded the Citizens Committee for the Conquest of Cancer when her husband Albert Lasker died from intestinal cancer in the early 1950s, was instrumental in promoting the introduction of the National Cancer Act of 1971 in the U.S. that was signed into law by then President Richard Nixon. This landmark federal legislation initiated the national "War Against Cancer," which has spurred the development of important health organizations (such as the National Cancer Institute of the National Institutes of Health in the U.S.), the expenditure of billions of dollars of federal funding for important cancer research, the development of new cancer treatment strategies and medications, as well as the establishment of myriad new programs to support cancer prevention and control. However, it must be noted that it was not easy for individual advocates or their health advocacy organizations to accomplish such sweeping

influences on public health policies. It took concerted strategic communication efforts, including the development of effective media relations programs, fundraising efforts, lobbying strategies, and the establishment of powerful public/private partnerships to achieve these important health promotion goals.

The Communication Demands for Effective Health Advocacy

Evidence suggests that both individual PHAs and organizational HAGOs have the potential to use health advocacy to help address many of the health problems that elderly health care consumers confront if they can meet the strategic communication demands of effective health advocacy (Kreps, 2013; Parvanta, Nelson, & Harner, 2017; Servaes & Malikhao, 2010). PHAs typically use strategic interpersonal communication to support the health needs of individual patients and families, although they also often communicate with groups (such as health care teams) and organizations (such as insurance companies) to achieve advocacy goals (Kreps, 2013). HAGOs also use different media channels and technologies strategically to represent the needs of groups of health care consumers, typically on organizational and even societal levels to achieve advocacy goals (Kreps & Kim, 2013). These individual and organizational health advocacy activities can help to recalibrate the traditional imbalance of power in health care and health promotion efforts as a powerful social mechanism for supporting consumer-driven participation and change within health care systems (Kahana et al.,2018; Kim, 2007; Moss, 2017; Teague et al.,2019).

Health advocates (both on the individual and organizational levels) also depend on strategic interpersonal communication to achieve their advocacy goals. Individual level and organizational level health advocates must learn how to actively represent the voices, concerns, and needs of the consumers they represent within the health care system (Kreps, 2013). This means establishing meaningful and trusting interpersonal communication relationships with the individual patients who advocates represent, to learn about these patients' unique goals, expectations, and concerns, as well as to learn about the best ways to communicate relevant health information to specific patients to promote high levels of health information comprehension and informed decision making (Kreps, 2012; 2013; 2018). Advocates also have great opportunities to help make health care programs responsive and adaptive to consumer needs through strategic health communication with health care providers, heath system administrators, and policy makers (Kreps et al., 2012; 2013). For example, strategic health advocacy communication can be used to help promote important influences on the development and refinement of important health policies and practices. To achieve their policy goals, health advocates strive to communicate patients' perspectives and needs in compelling ways to key audiences using a variety of different communication channels and media to influence often entrenched

health policies and practices (Kreps, 1996; 2013).

Sharing Relevant Health Information

Communication is at the center of effective health care and health promotion with elderly patients, because communication provides elderly consumers and their health care providers with the relevant health information that these health care system participants need to generate the best care and make their best health decisions (Kreps, 1988). Relevant and timely health information is a critical resource in health care and health promotion because it is used to guide health care provider decisions about diagnosis and treatment, as well as by elderly health care consumers to help them make important informed choices concerning preventing health risks, promoting their health, and for selecting their best health care treatments. Health information includes the knowledge gleaned from health care interviews and laboratory tests used to diagnose health problems, the precedents developed through clinical research and practice used to determine the best available treatment strategies for specific health threats, the data gathered in checkups used to assess the efficacy of health care treatments, the input practitioners and consumers need to evaluate bioethical issues and weigh consequences in making complex health care decisions, the recognition of warning signs needed to detect imminent health risks and to encourage adoption of health behaviors to help avoid these risks. Health care providers and consumers depend on their abilities to communicate effectively to generate, access, and exchange relevant health information for making important treatment decisions, for adjusting to changing health conditions, and for coordinating health-preserving activities. The use of strategic, evidence-based communication also enables effective dissemination of relevant and persuasive information appropriate to specific patients, providers, and other key audiences to influence health knowledge, attitudes, and behaviors. Health advocacy communication activities support the critically important health information needs for elderly health care consumers and for their caregivers.

Access to and effective use of relevant, accurate, and timely health information is essential for guiding the important health-related decisions that elderly health care consumers and their formal and information caregivers must make across the continuum of care (including the important interrelated care stages of Prevention, Detection, Diagnosis, Treatment, Survivorship, and End-of-Life) to promote health and well-being (Kreps, 2003; Kreps & Sivaram, 2010). This includes guiding decisions about the prevention of health risks, health promotion behaviors, the detection and diagnosis of health problems, health care treatment strategies, and best practices for living with health threats (successful survivorship) (Kreps, 2003). Yet health information is often exceedingly complex, with many different health risks, each with different causes, stages, symptoms, detection processes, and treatment strategies.

Health care knowledge is also rapidly evolving with advances in research and applications concerning the unique etiology, prevention, detection, diagnosis, and treatment of health problems for the elderly. It is extremely difficult for elderly health care consumers, as well as for many health care providers, to stay abreast of all the health information they need to make their best health decisions. They need support to manage the complex and evolving health information environment. Health advocates are essential for helping to assist with gathering, interpreting, and applying relevant health information (Kreps, 2013).

A primary goal of health advocacy organizations is to help break through the complexity of health and health care by disseminating relevant, timely, accurate, and clear health information to consumers and providers to help guide informed health decision making. However, there are significant barriers to the effective dissemination of health information, especially for elderly at-risk populations, due to problems they often have that limit their access to health information based upon health literacy challenges they often face, limited education levels, and the complexity of health research and health care processes (Kreps 2012; 2006; Wen et al., 2010). Health advocates must develop strategic communication programs for gathering relevant health information, interpreting that information, and presenting the information in meaningful ways to those health care participants who most need that information for guiding important health decisions.

Using Communication to Navigate the Modern Heath Care System

Health advocates must be able to demystify the medical jargon, complex structures, and bureaucratic processes that have developed over-time for delivering care and promoting health in the modern world that can be confusing and frustrating for many elderly health care consumers (Kreps, 2013). These complex health system structures are likely to operate quite differently from one location to another, particularly across different health care facilities and in different locations. Advocates must learn about local norms, regulations, and jargon wherever they are providing advocacy support so they can provide the best advice. Effective advocacy demands the ability to collect information and adapt communication practices to the different ways that health care delivery systems are organized and managed, the ways that health care services are financed, the ways that relevant treatments, medications, and technologies are developed, tested, and implemented, the ways that research programs are conducted to study health care and the promotion of health, as well as the ways that regulatory mechanisms and guidelines for governing the delivery of care are implemented (Kreps et al., 2012; 2013).

The complexities of modern health care systems often demands that health advocates for elderly consumers must be able to gather a great deal of complex information about a broad range of different health care systems and practices. They must learn about a wide range of different relevant health industries, including health care delivery systems, pharmaceutical companies, insurance organizations, and medical technology and supply industries. They need to learn about the many local, regional, and national government agencies that regulate heath care. They need to understand the ways that research programs are conducted to study health care tools, treatments, and processes. Moreover, they must learn the best ways to communicate with representatives of these different interrelated health care systems to promote cooperation and partnerships for refining health care practices and policies for elderly patients. In addition, health advocates need to understand the best ways to disseminate relevant information about the health care system to key audiences, particularly in reference to specific elderly health consumers' needs and concerns. There is clearly a lot of information for health care advocates to gather and make sense of, as well as to strategically communicate to key audience to effectively advocate for meeting the health needs of elderly consumers!

Interpersonal Communication Competencies for Health Advocacy

Health advocates depend upon engaging in effective interpersonal communication to develop meaningful and cooperative health advocacy relationships with elderly patients, their HSOs, health care providers, administrators, and many others to achieve their advocacy goals (Kreps, 2013). Health advocates cannot possibly accomplish the complex goals of influencing health care policies and practices to support the needs of elderly health care consumers all by themselves. They need to use strategic communication partnerships to actively encourage a range of key individuals, including patients, health care providers and administrators, policy makers, and volunteers, to collaborate in sharing advocacy messages and supporting advocacy causes. In addition, advocacy group leaders need to motivate, train, direct, and supervise these key individuals to ensure they work effectively and cooperatively to achieve advocacy goals. The demand for health advocates to use well-honed relational communication skills to coordinate advocacy efforts is illustrated well in predictions proposed by the Relational Health Communication Competency Model (RHCCM) that postulates that the use of competent interpersonal communication among interdependent participants in health care systems can promote needed cooperation for achieving important health goals (Kreps, 1988; 2014; Query & Kreps, 1996). The predictions from this model about the powerful influences of relational communication on achieving health outcomes also suggest that competent and adaptive interpersonal communication skills are needed to build meaningful health relationships, share relevant health information, motivate cooperation, and influence behaviors to achieve health advocacy goals (Kreps, 2013; Kreps et al., 2012). Therefore, it is critically important to help health advocates and the elderly consumers they serve learn how to communicate effectively interpersonally to build cooperative health relationships.

Utilizing Media Effectively for Health Advocacy

Popular media (news, entertainment, and social media) are primary tools for disseminating relevant health information concerning the health needs and issues affecting groups of elderly health care consumers. The right media coverage using the best media channels can be instrumental in helping advocates reach and influence key audiences (Gallant et al., 2011; Houston Staples, 2009; Stellefson, Paige, Chaney, & Chaney, 2020; Wittet et al., 2017). For example, advocates can use popular media to reach people who are concerned about the issues relevant to effective care for elderly patients to encourage these audience members to serve as potential advocacy group members and volunteers. They may need to reach potential donors to generate financial and material support for advocacy efforts. They may also need to use the media to motivate public support for relevant legislation and policies, as well as to encourage support from key public officials. However, it is not easy to control media messages and media coverage. Strategic communication partnerships and carefully designed messaging is needed to promote cooperation between media producers and health advocates.

The most direct way to control media coverage would be for advocacy organization leaders to purchase media spots and advertising. Unfortunately, this can be very expensive, especially when paying for the use of dramatic and popular entertainment media, particularly television and film time, and to a lesser extent radio time. Another strategy for getting media coverage of issues relevant to elderly health care consumers is for advocacy organization leaders to seek free coverage by presenting advocacy messages as relevant news items. For example, advocacy leaders might submit public service announcements to media outlets for free dissemination. Unfortunately, public service announcements, even when accepted for presentation, rarely gain much exposure because they are typically programed for inexpensive (low viewership) presentation time periods. It is much more cost effective for health advocacy leaders to encourage free news media coverage of issues relevant to elderly health care consumers by earning it through the use of media advocacy to persuade media representatives to cover advocacy issues (Dorfman, Wallack, & Woodruff, 2005; Wallack et al., 1993).

Media advocacy is an intricate communication strategy to motivate mass media representatives to cover key stories that enhance the visibility and legitimacy of health advocacy organizations issues by pitching stories that are relevant, timely, dramatic, and attractive to these media representatives because these stories promise to appeal to key audiences. In essence, advocates try to create newsworthy messages concerning health issues of concern to elderly consumers that media representatives will want to cover as relevant and interesting stories. By building cooperative relationships with media representatives, staging newsworthy events, linking advocacy group issues to breaking news or existing stories, as well as by providing compelling editorial pieces and commentary on relevant issues, health advocates can encourage media coverage of advocacy policy issues that are especially relevant to elderly consumers, such as stories about access to needed and effective care, new and affordable treatments and medications, home health care services, long-term care needs, mental health needs and services, and the need for rehabilitation equipment and services (Applebaum et al., 2020; de Carvalho et al., 2017; Kahana, 2020). (All of these important elder health topics have been covered by media news channels during the COVID-19 pandemic).

Advocates can also encourage media advocacy coverage by preparing relevant story summaries, press releases, and media kits for media representatives that make it easy for these representatives to cover the advocacy group stories (Houston Staples, 2009). They can provide succinct and persuasive summaries of advocacy organizations' positions of key public issues. They can distribute relevant fact sheets that provide compelling data and evidence in support of key issues they want covered. They can provide interesting press releases, with names and contact information of potential sources for the stories. They can also provide relevant background articles to media representatives, as well as providing clear and compelling background information about the advocacy organization.

By encouraging voluntary media coverage, health advocates hope to encourage key support for the health advocacy of elderly consumers. The goal is to use free media coverage to influence and shape public debate, put pressure on policy makers, and encourage community support for the consumers' key issues. Media coverage can help set the public agenda concerning health advocacy concerns by raising awareness about key elder care issues, encouraging public discussion of these issues, and influencing private conversations about the issues to motivate support for social change (Wallack, et al., 1999).

Building cooperative collaborations with media representatives (in accordance with the postulates of the RHCCM) is critically important for motivating effective media coverage of health advocacy issues (Kreps, 2014). There are several key questions that health advocates need to be able to answer to attract media coverage of health advocacy issues. These include: Who are the media representatives for the media outlets that advocates want to cover important health advocacy issues? Are the messages they want covered right for the specific medium selected? Who are the audiences these media channels serve? What kinds of stories do these media outlets want to cover? What problems do advocates want to have addressed by the media? What are the ideal solutions to these problems? Who has the power to address these issues to promote relevant social change? What messages would convince these key audiences to act on these issues? Do the media messages that advocates want covered have "news value" for the audiences the media outlets serve? How can stories be pitched effectively to key media outlets? Can advocates help media representatives cover these stories well? Are requests for media coverage responsive to the many constraints that media systems face (such as media time/space available for presenting stories, the topics media outlets prefer to cover, the appropriate complexity of stories for audiences, including both ideas, visuals, and language used)? This means that advocates must pitch stories that are appropriate for specific media and the audiences they serve. Advocates need to provide media outlets with good visuals, soundbites, and/or compelling personal testimony to humanize the stories. To utilize media channels effectively, health advocacy leaders must be able to design compelling messages and encourage media support for disseminating relevant elder health messages to key audiences.

An increasingly important channel for communicating health advocacy messages relevant to the needs of elderly consumers is the use of digital, social, and e-health media (Stellefson et al., 2020). For example, websites have become a ubiquitous and pervasive part of the communication mix for health advocacy organizations (Gallant, Irizarry, & Kreps, 2007). The website is critical in helping to establish an identity for the advocacy organization and it is also can serve as a primary portal for communication with key constituents if it is designed to be interactive and easy to utilize. Unfortunately, too many health organization websites do not effectively utilize strategic interactive e-health communication features and fail to maximize communication with key audiences (Kreps & Neuhauser, 2010). Many health websites fail to be particularly interactive, engaging, or dynamic (Gallant et al., 2011). These e-health problems are particularly challenging for many elderly health care consumers, who may not have well-developed digital communication competencies (Song & Shin, 2020). To be effective, digital health programs must be designed to leverage the abilities of digital media to communicate vividly, interactively, and adaptively for different populations of users through the use of specially designed mobile and interactive applications, video, tailored message systems, message boards, social media, digital training, and user support systems (Kreps, 2000; 2017; Kreps & Neuhauser, 2010). For example, the use of tailored information systems, with messages that reflect the unique interests and backgrounds of different individuals, can allow health advocates to adapt online communication to meet unique needs, interests, orientations, and backgrounds of different audiences, ensuring that online communication is personal and relevant to meet the information needs and digital literacy skills of users (Kreps, 2000).

The website has morphed in recent years from being a mere repository of health information to being a portal to a range of exciting communication opportunities to connect, inform, and engage constituents of health advocacy groups (Kreps, 2017). For example, health advocacy websites can be designed as an entry point for access to online support groups, discussion boards, webinars, news feeds, and social media for elderly consumers and their caregivers. Online support groups have become a staple health communication medium for many health advocacy organizations, enabling constituents who are confronting challenging health issues to connect with others confronting similar challenges to exchange ideas and to provide needed social support (Kreps, 2017). Online support groups have become an important source of contact and interpersonal communication for many isolated elderly individuals, especially during the COVID-19 pandemic (Armitage & Nellums, 2020). Evidence suggests that online support groups can be even more effective for supporting the information and support needs of health care consumers than in-person support groups because they afford group members greater freedom to connect when they are in need, eliminate the need for travel to participate in the support group, and afford support group members a higher level of privacy and anonymity than in-person support groups (Wright, 2016). Perhaps one of the greatest opportunities to health advocacy organizations is to leverage the use of digital media to promote collaborations, through the sharing of relevant information and the building of social action partnerships to promote change (Neuhauser & Kreps, 2010). As technology advances, there will be increasing opportunities to adopt new and powerful digital communication applications to promote the use of strategic communication to achieve the goals of health advocacy for elderly health care consumers and for their caregivers.

The Demand for Health Advocacy Programs and Policies

Health advocates serve a vitally important role for representing the needs of elderly health consumers within the modern health care system, refining relevant public policies, and improving quality of care and the promotion of health. However, effective health advocacy depends on the strategic use of health communication to gather relevant health information and to disseminate key information to important audiences in ways that will motivate cooperation and support for health advocacy policies and programs. Effective advocacy demands effective health communication to elicit cooperation, gather and share relevant health information, adapt to complex health settings, and utilize media to disseminate information to key audiences.

Health Advocacy Training Programs

Health advocacy training programs have been developed that show promise for promoting the development of effective health advocacy communications skills and competencies. Several universities now offer certificates or graduate degree programs in health advocacy, including Johns Hopkins University, Assumption University, Sarah Lawrence College, the University of Illinois at Chicago, and the University

of Wisconsin. Several non-profit organizations also offer health advocacy training. An example of an advocacy training program that focuses on the development of relevant strategic communication advocacy competencies is the Global Advocacy Leadership Academy (GALA) that provides no-cost online and in-person training for health advocacy group leaders (Kreps & Kim, 2013; Kreps et al., 2012; 2013). The GALA training program adapts communication education to the unique advocacy environments in different health care settings and countries, working adaptively with health advocates to address their specific advocacy challenges (Kreps & Kim, 2013). Similarly, in recent years a number of important advocacy training programs have been developed to help health care professionals develop the communication skills needed to be effective health advocates (Blenner, Lang, & Prelip, 2017; Godinho, Murthy, & Ciraj, 2017; Masai et al., 2017; Soklaridis et al., 2018).

Organizations That Promote a Culture of Health Advocacy

Relevant programs and policies are also needed to support health advocacy activities and encourage adoption of a strong culture of health advocacy within the modern health care system. This is being accomplished by a variety of different organizations that provide health advocacy promoting programs and activities. For example, Thomas (2019) describes the efforts by the professional organization for health educators, the Society for Public Health Education (SOPHE), to hold health advocacy summits that encourage research, education, and outreach activities relevant to increasing understanding, conducting research, sharing information, and initiating health advocacy projects to mobilize the next generation of health advocates. This kind of professional activity helps to promote recognition about the importance of health advocacy and helps to recruit professionals to participate in health advocacy activities.

Similarly, the Patient Advocacy Foundation (PAF) is a national non-profit organization that helps to promote a strong culture of health advocacy, both by providing health advocacy case management services and financial aid to Americans with chronic, life-threatening, and debilitating illnesses, and through its sister organization the National Patient Advocate Foundation (NPAF) which advocates for policy solutions to common problems facing patients concerning health care access and affordability (Patient Advocacy Foundation, 2020). In addition, the PAF and the NPAF provide health advocacy information and education through its websites, publications, webinars, and meetings.

The National Association of Healthcare Advocacy (NAHAC) is another non-profit organization that has helped to promote a culture of health advocacy by establishing a community composed of practicing health advocates and those interested in learning about health advocacy to promote professional development of health advocates, advance the field of health advocacy, empower consumers to nav-igate the health care system effectively, influence public policies in support of patient-centered care, and to serve as a clearinghouse to help consumers locate health advocates through there National Directory of Healthcare Advocacy. The NAHAC holds conferences, educational roundtables, and networking activities for health advocates and have established best practices for health advocacy (National Association of Healthcare Advocacy, 2020).

The American Public Health Association (APHA) is a professional organization for public health scholars and practitioners that has been very active in addressing health advocacy policy issues as a primary voice for public health advocacy to ensure access to care, protect funding for core public health programs and services, and eliminate health disparities (American Public Health Association, 2020). The APHA works on health policy advocacy primarily by conducting health advocacy campaign activities, lobbying legislators, disseminating legislation action alerts and APHA policy statements, and by hosting APHA legislative and advocacy priorities update webinars.

Several health care delivery systems have introduced health advocacy services for their patients, especially for elderly patients who often need assistance, using patient navigators (Freeman, 2006), hospital chaplains (Teague et al., 2019), nurses (Abbasinia, Ahmadi, & Kazemnejad, 2020), and physicians (Luft, 2017) as patient advocates, resulting in improved health outcomes. For example, Harold Freeman (2006) famously introduced the nation's first patient navigator program at Harlem Hospital in New York City in 1990, which was so successful that it served as a model for the Patient Navigator Outreach and Chronic Disease Prevention Act signed into law by President Bush in 2005. The Harlem Patient Navigator Program was designed to help poor Black patients, often elderly Black patients, access needed cancer screening and care, resulting in significantly improved health outcomes for early detection of cancer and reductions in both morbidity and mortality for both breast cancer and colon cancer (Freeman, 2006; Freeman & Rodriquez, 2011). These programs show that hospital-based health advocacy services are effective and should be expanded for vulnerable patients! These hospital-based programs are most appropriate for use with older patients who may need help negotiating complex health care system due to infirmity, co-morbid health conditions, and/or health literacy challenges (Kreps, 1986; 1990;).

There is great need and potential for additional efforts to promote health advocacy education, practice, and policy to establish a strong and well-established societal culture for health advocacy for elderly health care consumers. We appear to be building momentum through the health advocacy efforts of a variety of professional associations, non-profit organizations, educational institutions, and health care delivery systems to support competent health advocacy services to enhance consumer access to and participation in health care for improving health outcomes. Health advocacy programs and policies are warranted to support the health care needs of elderly health care consumers who often need support in negotiating the modern health care system to achieve their health care goals.

References

Abbasinia, M., Ahmadi, F., & Kazemnejad, A. (2020). Patient advocacy in nursing: A concept analysis. *Nursing Ethics, 27*(1), 141-151.

Adelman, R. D., Greene, M. G., & Silva, M. D. (2017). Communication challenges with the elderly. Oxford Textbook of Communication in Oncology and Palliative Care, 334.

American Public Health Association. (2020). Policy statements and advocacy. https://www.apha.org/policies-and-advocacy (Accessed 8/10/2020).

Anisimov, V. N. (2020). Aging and cancer biology. *Geriatric Oncology, 32*(24) 91-109.

Applebaum, R., Nelson, M, Strake, J.K., & Kennedy, K. (2020). Policy does matter: Changing an unchangeable long-term care services system. *Journal of Elder Policy, 1*(1), 21-38.

Armitage, R., & Nellums, L. B. (2020). COVID-19 and the consequences of isolating the elderly. *The Lancet Public Health, 5*(5), e256.

Ayalon, L., Chasteen, A., Diehl, M., Levy, B., Neupert, S. D., Rothermund, K., Clemens, T. R., & Wahl, H. W. (2020). Aging in times of the COVID-19 pandemic: Avoiding ageism and fostering intergenerational solidarity. *Journal of Gerontology: Series B, Psychological Science Social Science.* (Online only) doi:10.1093/geronb/gbaa051

Banerjee, D., D'Cruz, M. M., & Rao, T. S. (2020). Coronavirus disease 2019 and the elderly: Focus on psychosocial well-being, ageism, and abuse prevention– An advocacy review. *Journal of Geriatric Mental Health, 7*(1), 4-10.

Beard, J. R., Officer, A., De Carvalho, I. A., Sadana, R., Pot, A. M., Michel, J. P., Sherlock, P.L., Epping-Jordan, J. E., Peeters, G. M., Mahanani, W. R., Thiyagarajan, J. A., & Chatterji, S. (2016). The World report on ageing and health: A policy framework for healthy ageing. *The Lancet, 387*(10033), 2145-2154.

Bell, J. F., Whitney, R. L., & Young, H. M. (2019). Family caregiving in serious illness in the United States: Recommendations to support an invisible workforce. *Journal of the American Geriatrics Society, 67*(S2), S451-S456.

Berger, J. T. (2020). Marginally represented patients and the moral authority of surrogates. *The American Journal of Bioethics, 20*(2), 44-48.

Blenner, S. R., Lang, C. M., & Prelip, M. L. (2017). Shifting the culture around public health advocacy: Training future public health professionals to be effective agents of change. *Health Promotion Practice, 18*(6), 785-788.

Blyskal, J. (2020, June 17). *Loved one sick with covid-19? A patient advocate can help.* The Washington Post. https://www.washingtonpost.com/life style/wellness/loved-one-sick-with-covid-19-a-patient-advocate-can help/2020/06/15/9a1d9af4-a4f0-11ea-b473-04905b1af82b_story.html

Cheng, Y., Goodin, A. J., Pahor, M., Manini, T., & Brown, J. D. (2020). Healthcare utilization and physical functioning in older adults in the United States. *Journal of the American Geriatrics Society, 68*(2), 266-271.

Colenda, C. C., Reynolds, C. F., Applegate, W. B., Sloane, P. D., Zimmerman, S., Newman, A. B., Meeks, S., & Ouslander, J. G. (2020). COVID-19 Pandemic and Ageism: A Call for Humanitarian Care. *American Journal of Geriatric Psychiatry, 28*(8), 805-807.

Conrad, E. J., Becker, M., Brandley, E., Saksvig, E., & Nickelson, J. (2019). Advocacy and Public Policy Perceptions and Involvement of College Health Promotion Students. *Health Promotion Practice, 20*(5), 730-741.

D'Cruz, M., & Banerjee, D. (2020). 'An invisible human rights crisis': The marginalization of older adults during the COVID-19 pandemic–An advocacy review. *Psychiatry Research, 292*(113369), 1-9.

Darien, G. 2018. Transformation: My experience as a patient and an advocate in three chapters. NAM Perspectives. Commentary, National Academy of Medicine, Washington, DC. https://doi.org/10.31478/201810d.

de Carvalho, I. A., Epping-Jordan, J., Pot, A. M., Kelley, E., Toro, N., Thiyagarajan, J. A., & Beard, J. R. (2017). Organizing integrated health-care services to meet older people's needs. *Bulletin of the World Health Organization, 95*(11), 756-763.

Dillard, R. L., Perkins, M., Hart, A., Li, C., Wincek, R., Jones, D., & Hackney, M. E. (2018). Research advocacy training program benefits diverse older adults in participation, self-efficacy and attitudes toward research. *Progress in Community Health Partnerships: Research, Education, and Action, 12*(4), 367-380.

Dohan, D., & Schrag, D. (2005). Using navigators to improve care of underserved patients: current practices and approaches. *Cancer, 104*(4), 848–855.

Dorfman, L., Wallack, L., & Woodruff, K. (2005). More than a message: framing public health advocacy to change corporate practices. *Health Education & Behavior, 32*(3), 320-336.

Freeman, H. P. (2006). Patient navigation: A community-based strategy to reduce cancer disparities. *Journal of Urban Health, 83*(2), 139-141.

Freeman, H. P., & Rodriguez, R. L. (2011). History and principles of patient navigation. *Cancer, 117*(S15), 3537-3540.

Gallant, L. M., Irizarry, C., Boone, G. M., & Kreps, G. L. (2011). Promoting participatory medicine with social media: New media applications on hospital websites that enhance health education and e-patients' voice. *Journal of Participatory Medicine*, 3. http://www.jopm.org/evidence/research/2011/10/31/promoting-participatory-medicine-with-social-media-new-media-applications-on-hospital-websites-that-enhance-health-education-and-e-patients-voices/.

Gallant, L.M., Irizarry, C., & Kreps, G.L. (2007). User-centric hospital websites: A case for trust and personalization. *E-Service Journal, 5*(2), 5-26.

Godinho, M. A., Murthy, S., & Ciraj, A. M. (2017). Health policy for health professions students: building capacity for community advocacy in developing nations. *Education for Health, 30*(3), 254-255.

Gray, T. F., Nolan, M. T., Clayman, M. L., & Wenzel, J. A. (2019). The decision partner in healthcare decision-making: A concept analysis. *International Journal of Nursing Studies, 92,* 79-89.

Greenfield, S., Kaplan, S., & Ware, J. Jr. (1985). Expanding patient involvement in care: Effects on patient outcomes. *Annals of Internal Medicine, 102,* 520–528.

Harris, M., Bayer, A., & Tadd, W. (2002). Addressing the information needs of older patients. *Reviews in Clinical Gerontology, 12*(1), 5-11.

Hooker, K., Mejía, S. T., Phibbs, S., Tan, E. J., & Stevens, J. (2019). Effects of age discrimination on self-perceptions of aging and cancer risk behaviors. *The Gerontologist, 59*(Supplement_1), S28-S37.

Houston Staples, A. (2009). Media advocacy: A powerful tool for policy change. *North Carolina Medical Journal, 70*(2), 175-178.

Kahana, E. (2020). Introducing the Journal of Elder Policy during the Covid-19 pandemic: Why policies that protect older adults are more important than ever. *Journal of Elder Policy, 1*(1), 1-20.

Kahana, B., Yu, J., Kahana, E., & Langendoerfer, K. B. (2018). Whose advocacy counts in shaping elderly patients' satisfaction with physicians' care and communication? *Clinical Interventions in Aging, 13,* 1161-1168.

Kahana, E., Cheruvu, V. K., Kahana, B., Kelley-Moore, J., Sterns, S., Brown, J. A., & Stange, K. C. (2010). Patient advocacy and cancer screening in late life. *Open Longevity Science, 4,* 20-29.

Kahana, E., & Kahana, B. (2003). Patient proactivity enhancing doctor–patient–family communication in cancer prevention and care among the aged. *Patient Education and Counseling, 50*(1), 67-73.

Kinsella-Meier, M. A. (2019). How to best support families and caregivers who are disconnected, alienated, and underserved so they can become involved and effective advocates. *Odyssey: New Directions in Deaf Education, 20,* 34-38.

Kreps, G.L. (2018). Promoting patient comprehension of relevant health information. *Israel Journal of Health Policy Research, 7,* (56), 1-3 https://doi.org/10.1186/s13584-018-0250-z

Kreps, G.L. (2017). Online information and communication systems to enhance health outcomes through communication convergence. *Human Communication Research, 43*(4), 518-530. DOI: 10.1111/hcre.12117

Kreps, G.L. (2014). Relational health communication competence model. In T.L.

Thompson, (Ed.). *Encyclopedia of Health Communication, Volume III* (pp. 1160-1161), Los Angeles, CA: Sage Publications.

Kreps, G.L. (2013). Strategic communication for health advocacy and social change. In D. K. Kim, A. Singhal, and G.L. Kreps, (Eds.), *Health Communication: Strategies for Developing Global Health Programs* (pp. 281-296). New York: Peter Lang Publishers.

Kreps, G. L. (2012). Consumer control over and access to health information. *Annals of Family Medicine, 10*(5), 428-34.

Kreps, G.L. (2003). The impact of communication on cancer risk, incidence, morbidity, mortality, and quality of life. *Health Communication, 15*(2), *161-169.*

Kreps, G.L. (2000, November). The role of interactive technology in cancer communications interventions: Targeting key audience members by tailoring messages. Paper presented to the American Public Health Association annual conference, Boston.

Kreps, G.L. (1996). Communicating to promote justice in the modern health care system. *Journal of Health Communication*, 1(1), *99-109.*

Kreps, G.L. (1990). A systematic analysis of health communication with the aged. In H. Giles, N. Coupland, & J.M. Wiemann (Eds.), *Communication, health, and the elderly*, (pp. 135-154). Manchester, England: University of Manchester Press.

Kreps, G.L. (1988). The pervasive role of information in health and health care: Implications for health communication policy. *Annals of the International Communication Association, 11*(1), 238-276. Kreps, G.L. (1986). Health communication and the elderly. *World Communication, 15,* 55-70.

Kreps, G.L., & Chapelsky Massimilla, D. (2002). Cancer communications research and health outcomes: Review and challenge. *Communication Studies, 53*(4), *318-336.*

Kreps, G.L., & Kim, P. (2013). Using data to guide effective cancer advocacy group leadership training and support programs: The case of the Global Advocacy Leadership Academy (GALA). *Psycho-Oncology,* 22(S3), 135-136.

Kreps, G.L., Kim, P., Sparks, L., Neuhauser, L., Daugherty, C.G., Canzona, M.R., Kim, W., & Jun, J. (2013). Promoting effective health advocacy to promote global health: The case of the Global Advocacy Leadership Academy (GALA). *International Journal on Advances in Life Sciences, 5*(1 & 2), 66-78.

Kreps, G.L., Kim, P., Sparks, L., Neuhauser, L., Daugherty, C.G., Canzona, M.R., Kim, W., & Jun, J. (2012). Introducing the Global Advocacy Leadership

Academy (GALA): Training health advocates around the world to champion the needs of health care consumers. In G. L. Kreps, & P. Dini, (Eds.), *Global health 2012: The first international conference on global health challenges* (pp. 97-100). Wilmington, DE: International Academy, Research, and Industry Association (IARIA).

Kreps, G.L., & Neuhauser, L. (2010). New directions in e-health communication: Opportunities and challenges. *Patient Education and Counseling, 78,* 329-336.

Kreps, G. L., Neuhauser, L., Sparks, L., & Labelle, S. (2020). Promoting convergence between health literacy and health communication. *Studies in Health Technology and Informatics, 269,* 526-543, doi: 10.3233/SHTI200025.

Kreps, G. L., & O'Hair, D. (Eds.). (1995). *Communication and health outcome* Cresskill, NJ: Hampton Press.

Kreps, G. L., & Sivaram, R. (2010). The central role of strategic health communication in enhancing breast cancer outcomes across the continuum of care in limited-resource countries. *Cancer, 113*(S8), 2331-2337.

Leontiou, J. F. (2020). *The doctor still knows best: How medical culture is still marked by paternalism.* Peter Lang Publishing.

Levit, L. A., Singh, H., & Klepin, H. D. (2020). Cancer and aging activities at the American Society of Clinical Oncology and beyond: Reflections on the legacy of Dr. Arti Hurria. *Journal of Geriatric Oncology, 11*(2), 151-153.

Luft, L. M. (2017). The essential role of physician as advocate: how and why we pass it on. *Canadian Medical Education Journal, 8*(3), e109-e116.

Masai, L., Palma, G., Blenner, S., & Prelip, M. (2017, November). Advocacy training in public health: Giving students the tools to succeed. In APHA 2017 Annual Meeting & Expo (Nov. 4-Nov. 8). American Public Health Association.

Mattson, M., & Lam, C. (2015). *Health advocacy: A communication approach.* New York, NY: Peter-Lang.

Morgan Jr, R. C., & Reid, T. N. (2020). On Answering the Call to Action for COVID-19: Continuing a Bold Legacy of Health Advocacy. *Journal of the National Medical Association, 112*(6), 675-680. doi: 10.1016/j.jnma.2020.06.011

Natale-Pereira, A., Enard, K.R., Nevarez, L., & Jones. L.A. (2011). The role of patient navigators in eliminating health disparities. *Cancer, 117*(15), 3543-3552.

National Association of Healthcare Advocacy. (2020). *Guidance through the deep waters of today's healthcare.* https://www.nahac.com/#!event-list (Accessed 8/10/2020).

Parvanta, C., Nelson, D. E., & Harner, R. N. (2017). *Public health communication: Critical tools and strategies.* Jones & Bartlett Learning.

Patient Advocacy Foundation. (2020). *About us/our history.* https://www.patient advocate.org/learn-about-us/our-history/ (Accessed 8/10/2020).

Petronio, S., Sargent, J., Andea, L., Reganis, P., & Cichocki, D. (2004). Family and friends as healthcare advocates: Dilemmas of confidentiality and privacy. *Journal of Social and Personal Relationships, 21*(1), 33-52.

Query, J. L. & Kreps, G. L. (1996). Testing a relational model of health communication competence among caregivers for individuals with Alzheimer's disease. *Journal of Health Psychology, 1*(3), 335-352.

Schwartz, L. (2002). Is there an advocate in the house? The role of health care professionals in patient advocacy. *Journal of Medical Ethics, 28*(1), 37-40.

Servaes, J., & Malikhao, P. (2010). Advocacy strategies for health communication. *Public Relations Review, 36*(1), 42-49.

Sklar, D. P. (2016). Why effective health advocacy is so important today. *Academic Medicine, 91*(10), 1325-1328.

Soklaridis S, Bernard C, Ferguson G, Andermann L, Fefergrad M, Fung K, Iglar, K., Johnson, A., Paton, M., & Whitehead, C. (2018). Understanding health advocacy in family medicine and psychiatry curricula and practice: A qualitative study. *PLoS ONE 13*(5): e0197590. https://doi.org/ 10.1371/ journal.pone.0197590.

Song, J. H., & Shin, S. J. (2020). The effects of e-health literacy and subjective health status on health-seeking behaviors of elderly ising the Internet in the community. *Journal of Digital Convergence, 18*(1), 321-332.

Stellefson, M., Paige, S. R., Chaney, B. H., & Chaney, J. D. (2020). Evolving role of social media in health promotion: updated responsibilities for health education specialists. *International Journal of Environmental Research and Public Health, 17*(4), 1153, doi:10.3390/ijerph17041153.

Stewart, M., Meredith, L., Brown, J. B., & Galajda, J. (2000). The influence of older patient-physician communication on health and health-related outcomes. *Clinics in Geriatric Medicine, 16*(1), 25-36.

Street, R. L., Makoul, G., Arora, N. K., & Epstein, R. M. (2009). How does communication heal? Pathways linking clinician–patient communication to health outcomes. *Patient Education and Counseling, 74*(3), 295-301.

Sundler, A. J., Darcy, L., Råberus, A., & Holmström, I. K. (2020). Unmet health-care needs and human rights—A qualitative analysis of patients' complaints in light of the right to health and health care. *Health Expectations, 23,* 613-620. DOI: 10.1111/hex.13038.

Teague, P., Kraeuter, S., York, S., Scott, W., Furqan, M. M., & Zakaria, S. (2019). The role of the chaplain as a patient navigator and advocate for patients in the intensive care unit: one academic medical center's experience. *Journal of Religion and Health, 58*(5), 1833-1846.

Thomas, E. (2019). Mobilizing the next generation of health advocates: Building our collective capacity to advocate for health education and health equity through SOPHE Advocacy Summits. *Health Promotion Practice, 20*(1), 12-14.

Wallack, L., Woodruff, K., Dorfman, L., & Diaz, I. (1999). *News for a change: An advocate's guide to working with the media.* Thousand Oaks, CA: Sage Publications, Inc.

Wallack, L., Dorfman, L., Jernigan, D., & Themba, M. (1993). *Media advocacy and public health: Power for prevention.* Newbury Park, CA: Sage Publications, Inc.

Wright, K. (2016). Social networks, interpersonal social support, and health outcomes: A health communication perspective. *Frontiers in Communication, 1,* 1-6.

Wyman, M. F., Shiovitz-Ezra, S., & Bengel, J. (2018). Ageism in the health care system: Providers, patients, and systems. In L. Ayalon & C. Tesch-Römer (Eds.), *Contemporary perspectives on ageism* (pp. 193-212). Springer.

Aging in Prison and the Social Mirror: Reflections and Insights on Care and Justice

Tina Maschi, Ph.D., LCSW, ACSW[1*]

Keith Morgen, Ph.D., LPC, ACS[2]

Karen Bullock, Ph.D., LCSW[3]

Adriana Kaye, LMSW[1]

Annette M. Hintenach, MSSW[1]

[1] Professor, Fordham University, Graduate School of Social Service

[2] Centenary University, Social & Behavioral Sciences Department

[3] North Carolina State, School of Social Work

*Corresponding Author: tmaschi@fordam.edu

ABSTRACT

In the era of COVID-19, there is a growing awareness of what was once an "unseen problem" of the crisis of a rapidly growing population of the aged, sick, and dying who are behind lock and key. This article provides a global overview of the aging prison population as well as an in-depth analysis of select and salient existing community and policy responses to justice-involved older adults. Moving towards a more solution-focused and visionary approach to imagine an ideal society that would address social determinants of health, justice disparities, and the current "aging in prison" crisis is discussed. Based on three decades of research, practice research, and wisdom, a global shift from a competition and conflict societal approach to a caring justice model is proposed. Select programs of promising global practices that governmental and non-governmental organizations may use to guide their response to their populations that directly target the crisis of justice-involved older people, their families, and communities are presented. A reflective analysis applied to the aging prison population has relevance for other global communities grappling with similar complex issues regarding societal ills, poor health and early mortality, homelessness, unemployment, community violence, natural and human-made disaster, and mass incarceration of people of all ages.

Keywords: prison, prisoners, criminal justice, well-being, human rights, social justice, elder justice policy, compassionate care

doi: 10.18278/jep.1.2.6

El envejecimiento en la prisión y el espejo social: Reflexiones y perspectivas sobre el cuidado y la justicia

Resumen

En la era de COVID-19, existe una creciente conciencia de lo que alguna vez fue un "problema invisible" de la crisis de una población en rápido crecimiento de ancianos, enfermos y moribundos que están bajo llave. Este artículo proporciona una descripción general del envejecimiento de la población carcelaria, así como un análisis en profundidad de las respuestas políticas y comunitarias existentes seleccionadas y destacadas para los adultos mayores involucrados en la justicia. Se analiza el avance hacia un enfoque más visionario y centrado en soluciones para imaginar una sociedad ideal que aborde los determinantes sociales de la salud, las disparidades en la justicia y la actual crisis del "envejecimiento en prisión". Sobre la base de tres décadas de investigación, investigación práctica y sabiduría, se propone un cambio global de un enfoque social de competencia y conflicto a un modelo de justicia solidaria. Se presentan programas selectos de prácticas globales prometedoras que las organizaciones gubernamentales y no gubernamentales pueden utilizar para orientar su respuesta a sus poblaciones que se dirigen directamente a la crisis de las personas mayores involucradas en la justicia, sus familias y comunidades. Un análisis reflexivo aplicado al envejecimiento de la población carcelaria tiene relevancia para otras comunidades globales que luchan con problemas complejos similares con respecto a enfermedades sociales, mala salud y mortalidad temprana, falta de vivienda, desempleo, violencia comunitaria, desastres naturales y provocados por el hombre y encarcelamiento masivo de personas de todas las edades.

Palabras clave: prisión, presos, justicia penal, bienestar, derechos humanos, justicia social, política de justicia para personas mayores, atención compasiva

在监狱中老去和社会镜像：关于护理和正义的反思和见解

摘要

新冠肺炎（COVID-19）期间，监狱中快速增加的老龄、生病及死亡人口—这一曾是"看不见的问题"—得到越来越多的关注。本文从全球层面概述了监狱中的老龄人口，并深入分析了针对涉及刑事司法的老年人的、最佳的现有社区响应和政策响应。朝更聚焦于解决方案和前瞻性的方法发展，设想一个能应对"卫生差异和司法差异的社会决定因素"的理想社会，并探讨了当前的"在监狱中老去"危机。基于三十年的研究、实践研究和智慧，提出了一个从竞争和冲突的社会模式转变为一个关爱的正义模式的全球转型。展现了关于有希望的全球实践的最佳计划，政府和非政府组织能通过这些实践指导其对各自人口的响应，并且这些实践直接针对涉及刑事司法的老年人及其家庭和社区。对监狱老年人口使用的反思性分析对其他面临相似复杂问题的全球社区具有相关性，这些问题包括社会问题、身体虚弱和早期死亡、无家可归、失业、社区暴力、自然和人为灾害、以及各年龄段的大规模监禁。

关键词：监狱，囚犯，刑事司法，福祉，人权，社会正义，老年正义政策，人文关怀

We cannot solve our problems with the same level of thinking that created them.

—Albert Einstein

There is a growing awareness of what was once an "unseen problem": the crisis of a rapidly growing population of the aged, sick, and dying with special needs, who are behind lock and key. In the United States, the growth of the incarcerated aging population is alarming because prisons were not built to adapt to their unique needs. These prisons often lack the trained staff and medical resources that would make them qualified long-term health care facilities. This may include any type of restorative and rehabilitative health care services, as well as skilled nursing care, to assist aging prisoners with their activities of daily living. This think piece is guided by the meaning behind Einstein's quote: "*We cannot solve our problems with the same level of thinking that created them.*" It has the objective to take readers through the mountainous territory that led to the current critical point of the "aging-in-prison" crisis, confounded by the coronavirus inside prisons and in communities across the world. We invite readers to examine the miscellany of meanings that can be gleaned from this situation and assume multiple perspectives of seeing the world through the eyes of an older adult in prison, as well as the observer self as an actor in society.

Engaging various viewpoints and based on empirical evidence, we bring knowledge and wisdom of multiple key stakeholders and create a montage of the longitudinal and holistic psycho-social, structural portraits of members of the aging prison population. The data presented in this article comes from the Hartford Prison Study (HPS). The study was conducted in September 2010 in a northeastern state prison system, which consisted of fourteen prisons in which adults aged 50 and older may be housed. This study used a cross-sectional correlational design and self-administered mailed surveys. Of the approximately 25,000 adults housed in this state correctional facility in January 2010, approximately 7% (n=1,750) were aged 50 and older, of which 1,700 male and 50 were female. Information to create the sampling frame included the state numbers, prison location, and demographic information, such as age and gender. Invitations were mailed to all 1,750 potential older adults. A total of 677 surveys were returned and a 40% response rate was achieved. This estimate falls within the higher range of expected mail response rates, which are 20-40% for prison populations. A series of descriptive and advanced statistical and modeling methods have been used to analyze the research studies published on the Hartford Prison Study (Maschi et al., 2015).

This national and international recognition of cruel prison conditions has been reflected through many outlets, such as increased media coverage as well as increased attention in academic and professional newspapers and group conversations (Maschi & Kaye, 2018; New York Times, 2017). The images of diverse older adults, such as those shown here, together with their unique and collective life stories, before, during, and after prison, has brought local and global recognition of this fast-growing "silver tsunami" (Bartels & Naslund, 2013). Some of the issues that members of the older generation struggle with, particularly minority groups, are linked to early life cumulative disadvantages such as health and mental health problems, social isolation and inequality, toxic stress, prejudice, and lack of access to quality education, and community services (Maschi et al., 2013). Furthermore, the experiences of prolonged imprisonment significantly exacerbate these cumulative disadvantages (Maschi et al., 2011; Maschi et al., 2014; Maschi et al., 2015).

During the COVID-19 pandemic, we analyze the incarceration and community contexts of the current aging population of the global environment, from serving time in prison to post-prison release and community reintegration, as we contend with the global public health and public safety crises. During these crises, we see similar trajectories in communities that are hardest hit by the pandemic, including, but not limited to, predominantly Black and Latino communities in inner cities and rural areas (Benfer et al., 2020).

The paper is structured as follows: it begins with a brief global overview of the problem, followed by a more in-depth analysis of salient existing community and policy responses to justice-involved older adults. Next, we shift our thinking to a more solution-focused and visionary approach to imagine an ideal society that would address the social determinants of health and justice disparities and the current "aging in prison" crisis. Based on our three decades of research, practice research, and wisdom, we propose a global shift from a competition and conflict societal approach to a caring justice partnership (CJP) model. Next, we provide examples of existing policies and programs that are or could be integrated into society. We also present select programs of promising global practices that governmental and non-governmental organizations can use to guide their response to their populations that directly target the crisis of justice-involved older people and their families and communities. This reflective analysis applied to the aging in prison also has relevance for other global communities grappling with similar complex issues regarding societal ills, poor health and early mortality, homelessness, unemployment, community violence, natural and human-made disaster, and mass incarceration of people of all ages.

A Portrait of Older Adults in Prison

Older adults in prison have different pathways and timelines to and through prison. Some older adults may enter prison later in life. Others will return to prison one or more times for similar crimes or for parole violations, especially if they have mental health or substance abuse prob-

lems and lack access to necessary community reentry services (Baillargeon et al., 2009; Harding et al., 2017; Maschi, Morrisey, & Leigey, 2013).

We have classified incarcerated older adults with long-term or life sentences into three distinct groups: 1) the life course (prison) older adults, 2) acute and chronic recidivists, and 3) late-onset offenders (Maschi, Gibson, Zgoba, et al., 2011). In order to determine incarceration and criminal offense patterns, this article uses a modified version of Goetting's (1984) incarcerated older adult typography, a notable design for older prisoners' sentencing histories. This includes four sub-populations. Those are: 1) young short-term first offenders; 2) old timers; 3) career criminals; and 4) older offenders. Young short-term first-time offenders are juveniles or adults who have been incarcerated prior to older age and released prior to older age. The old timers are adult inmates who serve for 20 or more years and grow old while in prison. Career criminals are recidivists (not including old timers) who serve two or more prison terms for varying lengths of time, sometimes for older adults. Older offenders will first be imprisoned during older adulthood (Aday, 2003; Goetting, 1984; Maschi, Gibson, Zgoba, et al., 2011).

While older adults and the serious and terminally ill are considered a special needs population in prison (UNODC, 2009), at opposite ends of the age spectrum, there are imprisoned younger age groups who have different developmental needs as they age in and out of prison. For example, individuals who were incarcerated at a younger age, especially between ages of 18 to 24 years, enter prison during a critical developmental stage from late adolescence to early adulthood and must adapt to a highly stressful prison environment (West & Sabol, 2008). As incarcerated individuals reach older age in prison, their increased frailty often plagues them prematurely with more age-related, severe health and mental health issues, including increased risk for dementia (Maschi & Aday, 2014; Maschi et al., 2012; Shimkus 2004).

As for anomalies in health statuses, people aging in prison often have an accelerated aging process. In other words, the average incarcerated individual might experience accelerated decrements in their health equivalent to adults living in the community who are 15 years older (Codd, 2013; HRW, 2012; Maschi et al., 2012). The accelerated aging process is corroborated by evidence from international prison studies. They show that older incarcerated adults have significantly higher rates of physical and mental health decline compared to older adults' counterparts in the community (Dai & Yu, 2011; HRW, 2012). This rapid decline of incarcerated older adults' health has been attributed mainly to their high-risk personal histories, chronic health conditions, poor health practices, such as poor diets and smoking, alcohol and substance abuse, coupled with the stressful conditions of prison confinement, such as prolonged exposure to overcrowding, social isolation and deprivation, sedentary lifestyle and poor nutrition, and prison violence (Maschi et al., 2011; Stojkovic, 2007; UNODC, 2009; Williams et al., 2012). These collective personal, social, and environmental risk factors significantly increase the likelihood of the early onset of severe physical and mental illnesses, including dementia among older adults in prison (Maschi et al., 2011; Maschi et al., 2012; Williams et al., 2012).

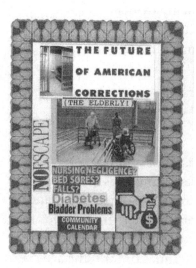

Figure 1. Worst Place on Earth, The Future of American Corrections: A Collage made by Ojore (created while he was incarcerated)

Below are two quotes of a prison hospice volunteer that exemplify the portrait of older adults in prison:

"The apathy of the guards toward dying inmates was unconscionable. We had one inmate about 30 years old whose wife and two small children were permitted a special visit because he was near death. As shift change approached, a nurse entered the room, and the family had to stand outside of the door. A female guard yelled to the nurse, 'Isn't he dead yet? I don't want to have to stay late to do the paperwork.' The two little girls were sobbing in no time."

—Joseph, a 57-year-old incarcerated man.

"We also had an inmate turn 100 years old there. He was completely bed-ridden. He eventually passed away. I was left wondering how society was being served by that. In the six months that I worked there, 6-7 inmates passed away. Hepatitis and diabetes cases abounded, with many amputations."

—Joseph, a 57-year-old incarcerated man.

Towards a Caring Justice Approach: Re-Calibrating the Fabric of Compassion and Justice Throughout Society

"Our human compassion binds us the one to the other—not in pity or patronizingly, but as human beings who have learnt how to turn our common suffering into hope for the future."

—Nelson Mandela

"True peace is not merely the absence of war; it is the presence of justice."

—Jane Addams

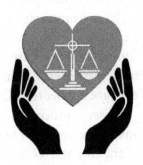

Older adults in prison shared their care experiences with us before and during imprisonment, and in anticipation of release. In these accounts, they shared the characteristics of treatment that fall below or above the level of good enough "care." Descriptions of their experiences obtained from families, societies, and prisons depicted circumstances that were often below acceptable standards of quality care and respect. Typically, there was a skewed display of power, violence and coercion, excessive use of force, intentional and unintentional negligence, dishonesty, deception, bullying tactics, narcissistic self-centeredness, arrogance, and recklessness from others. Several older adults shared that sometimes they felt degraded, oppressed, guilty, powerless, fearful, and shamed by formal and informal caregivers (Maschi & Morgen, 2020).

Readers should remember that listening to or hearing about trauma can have a detrimental effect on listeners. For example, the mere fact of watching television and the negative news stories makes us secondary witnesses to traumatic experiences such as pandemic COVID-19, domestic violence, street crime, and terrorism. Because of a mixture of negative interactions in different social environments (e.g., family home, culture, or service settings), certain criminal activities are activated and driven by strong emotions such as hatred, vengeance, rejection, or strong dogmatic values, cognitive distortions, or grandiose delusions. Hence, perhaps the fundamental core problems of complex injustice and bondage are the unidentified "dis-ease" of "lovesickness." And as the LGBT elders in jail told us, the cure is unconditional love and compassion from a loving person or people. The unconditional dimension of being welcomed despite who we are or what we did may be the cure. To better address these issues, having a nurturing atmosphere (as opposed to an unhealthy and punitive prison environment) will help in rehabilitating imprisoned older adults eligible for prison release. When it comes to parole consideration, many older adults are denied parole based on their history of violent criminal offense and may be expected to spend their lives in prison (Goetting, 1984; Maschi et al., 2013). As these are sensitive parole decisions, citizens should weigh in their views on how we could create a fair playing field among us by balancing care and justice for all concerned.

The "uncaring" behaviors that humans have conducted with each other and with their environments have reached epic proportions both in and out of prison. This old interpretation of our current social and environmental issues has gone its way. Therefore, we present a new way of understanding the same old problem and suggest a caring justice partnership (CJP) paradigm to tackle problems of care and justice. The foundation CJP model is one in which compassion and justice values are woven across the fabric of society and embedded in the individual, family, community, and the globe. We define the caring justice partnership paradigm as a regular philosophical practice or way of life intended to encourage personal and relational growth. Based on state-of-the-art physical and social sciences—physics, philosophy, psychology, and social work—we argue that we can address issues such as the aging in prison crisis if we shift from a problem-based focus to a solution-based focus. We explain how to use caring justice at the personal and collective levels and transform the world from within (Maschi & Morgen, 2020).

On the positive side, the older adults' accounts identified qualities of compassionate caregivers who helped them turn their lives around, such as valuing their dignity and life potential. When it comes to peer guidance, our research indicates the incarcerated older adults had a significant therapeutic effect on incarcerated younger individuals. When describing their experiences of compassionate informal and formal caregivers from the community or prisons, older adults reported that such individuals or agencies emanated unconditional love, dignity, worthiness, and respect. *"The staff there gave me genuine love and caring and respect. I walked out of there feeling at home and loved and worthy."* Authenticity, empathy, kindness, and unconditional love were other central values of compassionate caregivers (Maschi & Morgen, 2020).

Based on over a decade of our research on aging people in prison and service providers, the truthfulness and honesty that incarcerated elderly felt from compassionate caregivers laid the foundation for formal and informal therapeutic work relationships. Our data also showed that there was an experiential, emotional connection, that is, older adults viewed these providers as empathetic, caring, and non-judgmental and felt like they were receiving unconditional love. For example, one older adult with serious mental illness shared that he did not begin to retake his psychotropic medication until he had a compassionate psychiatrist. *"I had a compassionate psychiatrist who did not judge me and made me feel loved and safe even in prison."* It also became a pivotal moment for him to turn around his life, stop getting into fights, and take part in programs. Another quality of these caregivers is that they were communication skilled. They used verbal and non-verbal activities to build relationships with older adults (e.g., responding to them with dignity and respect, using active listening). Furthermore, such caregivers also had realistic, reliable, and solution-focused qualities. The older adults described them as hav-

ing responsibility and resourcefulness. Their helpful advice ranged from personal growth therapy to recommendations or lobbying for medications, programs, or resources they needed. In the expansion of their positive attitude and general well-being, being in the presence of a "loving" or caring person and learning to love and care about oneself was crucial in encouraging elderly incarcerated to change their lives (Maschi & Morgen, 2020).

Our community-based participatory research model has three general prompts. How can we co-construct communities for the welfare and wellness of all ages? What are the barriers and facilitators to the creation of a culture rooted in ideals of love, compassion, justice, and equality for all? What are the approaches suggested to remove barriers and promote the overall well-being of individuals, families, organizations, and communities? Communities can refer to the Co-constructing Community model for further guidance with this (Maschi & Koskinen, 2015).

Conceptualizing and Embodying Compassion and Justice

We propose recognizing the fundamental ethical values of compassion and justice, expressed by all individuals within a society. Compassion and justice as core concepts are specific, but complementary "patterns" of a caring partnership approach to justice. When we connect these two principles, compassion and justice, they carry unique strengths and promote the equilibrium of love, equality, and accountability.

First, there are multiple conceptualizations of compassion. A commonality among these definitions is the recognition, interpretation, and response to suffering in a nonjudgmental way (Gilbert, 2009). In eastern traditions, Buddhist teachings on compassion provide a way of interbeing that honors all living beings and demonstrates concern for alleviating the suffering of others. In other words, a compassionate person, family, party, organization, or society holds these principles at the heart of their work and purpose (Kordowicz, 2019). In the west, Paul Gilbert, the pioneer of compassion-focused therapy, clarifies that being compassionate includes opening oneself and others to suffering in a non-defensive and non-judgmental manner, a desire, and actions to relieve suffering (Gilbert, 2009).

Second, it is necessary to affirm justice in the framework of compassion, particularly as it relates to public safety, protection, and the foundation of essential human needs (Maschi et al., 2016). To understand the relationship between care and justice, we need to examine the history and significance of the concept of justice. The legal definition of justice in contemporary times has many variations inside itself. Justice in the United States is often defined as consistency of being just, impartial, or equitable, and being in conformity with reality, fact, or purpose and/or "maintenance or administration of what is just, by the impartial adjustment of

conflicting claims or the assignment of merited rewards or punishments" (Merriam-Webster, 2020).

On one hand, justice as a concept has been synonymous with fact, reason, equilibrium, order, harmony, rule, morality, ethics, fairness, equity, equality, law, faith, and justice across history, diverse cultures, and disciplines (Maschi et al., 2015; Maschi, Viola, & Koskinen, 2015). On the other hand, justice also often applies to opposites such as inequality, anarchy, the immorality of crime, differences, and negative behavior (LaLlave & Gutheil, 2012). Historically, the "injustices" of justice have been apparent, such as during the emergence of industrialization in the early 20th century, when the social aspects of justice and equality was of paramount importance, and the pursuit of "social and distributive justice" was advanced in social science disciplines. Procedural justice tried to understand the procedures and consequences in the analysis and application of the law and to strengthen the legal mechanisms that could ensure equality and fairness (Rawls & Kelly, 2003; Wakefield, 1988).

The caring justice global movement's goal is to change negative individual attitudes and behaviors into compassionate care for those at times of crisis and loss, including caretaking for the aging, seriously ill, and dying. These types of compassionate community models actively promote, facilitate, endorse, and celebrate care for one another during life's most testing moments and experiences. It uses an approach to community engagement and development, which seeks to connect, empower, and encourage "ordinary people to help ordinary people." A growing component of the model also emerges as the result of public discussions and community engagement from the grassroots. The development emphasis was on building community capacity through the creation and support of social networks, including peer and community support, particularly volunteers, with and for people of all ages. Applying this type of model to adult prisons, local communities, and policy practices at the local, national, and global levels will help to promote a more compassionate response to the criminal justice system, especially for the elderly, disabled, and dying in prison (Bunce, 2018). A kinder and gentler justice response has a higher probability of being more humane to the frail, sick, and dying compared to a punitive and retributive approach that we currently have. Policymakers must work together with other stakeholders to develop solutions for a more compassionate response at the local, national, and global levels.

After over a decade of research on trauma and the criminal justice systems with diverse age groups, we have found that many older adults face challenges in the physical, mental, financial, social, and spiritual realms (Maschi & Leibowitz, 2018). These studies have shown that that older adults in prison who use coping mechanisms that address those areas, will have better health relative to those who do not (Maschi, Dennis, Gibson, et al., 2011).

In our research, the coping resources older adults used fell within one or more of the following domains: root, physical, cognitive, emotional, social, spiritual, participatory, and multi-dimensional. While some older adults described their coping practices of well-being, other older adults felt appreciation for being able to meet their basic needs in prison. *"At least I have a cot."* Additionally, some older adults used physical coping resources, such as exercise or taking medication—*"I work out to relieve stress"* and *"I became a jogger and sprinter at 56 years old."* The older adults seemed to feel a sense of safety, security, and strength in reducing stress and increasing coping resilience using root and physical practices. Additionally, some older adults in prison also reported using cognitive coping strategies such as finding peace inside; making healthy decisions; reading books or other written materials; and playing games or mental exercises, such as puzzles. One incarcerated older adult found optimism and inner peace by meditating—*"I try to think positively and try to meditate and read a great deal to take my mind off worries."* Yet others have described emotional coping, often in the context of prison program offerings. Such activities included supportive emotional counseling and anger, and stress management. Certain activities that evoked emotional wellness included listening to music, writing/journaling, or engaging in play and pleasurable experiences. Social coping consisted of interactions with family, friends, peers in prison, and program participation. When it comes to spirituality, it was considered an internal and external expression of coping. Some focused on their inner connection with "God" and attended a religious service, while others thought of spirituality as praying and being of service to others. One older adult shared, *"I Pray to God and go to church regularly here."* Another older person practiced his spirituality by attending *"religious services, offer my prayers, and try as much as I can to be faithful to my oaths as a Muslim."* Participatory coping was described as self-empowerment and leadership. Several older adults were active in positions of leadership, taking classes or vocational training for personal advancement, coaching, running a book club, or activism in jail. Some activities were multidimensional and tapped multiple coping domains, such as art-making, music-making, and yoga. One older adult noted, *"I do yoga, doctor, I do yoga"* (Maschi & Morgen, 2020).

Various theories such as the life course perspective, stress process, and cumulative disadvantage theories complement the interdisciplinary and community-based approach to social determinants of health. They highlight how important and traumatic personal or historical life events impact the health and well-being of older adults in prison, society, and the interaction between them. They also emphasize the resilience or protective factors, such as internal and external coping mechanisms and services, which are essential to the development and maintenance of health and well-being and smooth transitions (Agnew, 1989; Elder, 1974, 2003; Laub & Sampson, 1993; Norris, 1992; Pearlin & Skaff, 1996; Sampson & Laub, 2003). Understanding that world-view of individuals and cultural groups influences how people make sense of health and well-being until the end of life (Maschi & Baer, 2013).

After all, these findings are validated by our body of research on trauma, coping, and well-being among older adults in prison (Maschi et al., 2015; Maschi, Viola, & Morgen, 2013). Our studies also have shown that older people who were engaged in biopsychosocial structural/spiritual coping activities, especially to reduce stress-related symptoms while in prison, reported higher levels of physical and mental well-being relative to those who did not. Indeed, our research indicates that older adults with a more positive view of themselves and others were less likely to report a history of recurrence and disciplinary offenses in prison compared to their counterparts who registered lower levels of coping skills. Such findings are consistent with empirical evidence that coping resources can buffer the adverse effects of traumatic life experiences on individuals' well-being (Maschi et al., 2015; Maschi, Dennis, Gibson, et al., 2011; Maschi, Viola, & Morgen, 2013).

The Gift of Life: Incarcerated Older Adults' Practices on Empowerment and Self-Care

In this segment, we demonstrate that, under the challenging conditions of confinement, older adults engage in naturally occurring self-care and empowerment activities that promote their health and well-being. Many participants mentioned interest in our studies to share their insights and experiences because they wanted to give the gift of life to others selflessly. We discuss self-care and empowerment behaviors that have been shown in quantitative and qualitative studies to enhance individual health, well-being, and healthy behaviors (Maschi & Morgen, 2020).

Maybe no one knows better than incarcerated older adults do about the value and preciousness of "life," particularly those with long term sentences. What do they tell us about life?

"Live life to the fullest. Love yourself more than love can love. You and you are all you need. You are beyond self-esteem; you are the 'esteemed' self. Choose to thrive despite the condition. Find a higher purpose and follow it upward. Be creative within confinement. Be the person in prison who sings. Be the person in the community who listens and sings back. Be the radiant glow and smell, and the single flower that happily grows in through a sidewalk crack. Let your sunshine and power your train in the positive light. Life is good." (Maschi & Morgen, 2020)

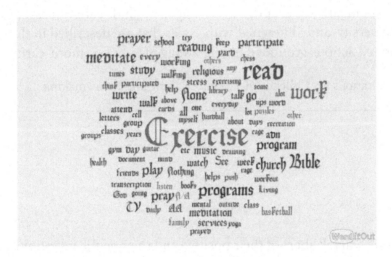

Figure 2. Word Cloud of Coping Resilience Activities
(Created from https://worditout.com/)

The *Accepting the Gift of Life,* a self-love-empowerment program, consists of various activities that older adults described and encouraged as beneficial to managing challenging conditions, such as stress in the prison environment or after their release. Contemplative practices may include meditation, yoga, creative arts, and reiki self-treatment, among other activities. They also promoted the implementation of organizational and community-level interventions. Such interventions are widespread may include everything from housing, health care, civic engagement, and trauma and community healing (Maschi & Morgen, 2020).

Trauma Healing Programs, Self, Organizations, and Communities

Ultimately, older adults in prison report that biopsychosocial/ structural/spiritual practices are a self-empowered prescription to living a long, happy, and healthy life despite their conditions. Our wise elders have urged us to a new way of approaching the gift of life. Humankind has always tested the human spirit. Yet the human spirit continuously ascends like the phoenix who rises from the fiery ashes of hatred and pain. Perhaps it is time to embark on a new way of "testing" diversity and difference with heart-centered actions grounded in un-conditional love and acceptance. Let us see how high the human spirit will usher in a caring justice world filled with peace, justice, honesty, and balance. We are humanity, and we thrive on expansion and growth. Let us see how high and long the phoenix can fly after it had the taste of swimming in waters of love. Now, that would be a new way of responding to the same old problem.

In the spirit of Einstein, *"We can't solve our problems with the same level of thinking that created them,"* we call for inspired action to implement a "New Age of Caring Justice" strategy and replace the Old Age of despair, apathy, and carelessness. The strategies that are described in the article are suggestive of a more caring and just

Table 1. Inspirations for Collective Decision-Making and Policymaking

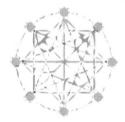

"Laws alone will fall short of their positive and therapeutic intentions unless they are fueled by the spirit of compassion in the entire population."
—Tina Maschi & Adriana Kaye

"Science deals mainly with facts; religion deals mainly with values. The two are not rivals." —Martin Luther King

"Justice that love gives is a surrender, justice that law gives is a punishment."
—Mahatma Gandhi

"Our task must be to free ourselves ... by widening our circle of compassion to embrace all living creatures and the whole of nature in its beauty."
—Albert Einstein

approach to collaborating and empowering people in prison or service uses and service providers. Basing the system more on compassion, as opposed to punishment and retribution, will not only assist in healthier and safer organizations and communities, but will empower individuals with the knowledge and skills to incorporate a daily affirmative life practice, such as the Gift of Life Program suggests.

A caring justice approach has the potential of liberating individuals and communities to consider replacing cruel and unusual punishment by mercy, compassion, unconditional love, transparency (truth), and accountability. Our old paradigm dies a good death with a fresh impetus and a new way of thinking. Ushering in a caring justice consciousness should direct the reform of the criminal justice system and help us prevent human-made public safety disasters, such as our prison systems. It can also help to take steps to provide emergency assistance to the aged, disabled, and dying in jail, as well as to members and groups of their families. A caring justice approach also suggests that "care"-ful analysis be conducted before responding. A holistic review will also encourage all key stakeholders in identifying the problems and crafting solutions collectively. In other words, a comprehensive analysis means that impulsive actions can be replaced with inspired actions. Table 1 offers several examples of motivating quotes indicative of what it might feel like to engage in motivated acts, as opposed to "knee jerk and impulsive reactions," taken

with only partial consideration of all the complexities of a question.

Currently, in the wake of COVID-19, we are at a crossroads where public concern is mounting. We can redefine this crisis as an opportunity to reinvent ourselves and our relationships with our families and communities.

Promising Compassionate Policies and Laws

If a CJP model was adopted, existing promising laws and practices might be practiced in some of these critical policies that directly target the older prison population. In some countries, compassionate policies and regulations can evidence some of the UN guidelines that affect aging prisoners. The United States, for example, has federal and state laws, mostly relating to incarcerated care as well as re-entry due to compulsory parole, detention, or medical or compassionate release policies (Chiu, 2010).

Since 2009, geriatric release requirements in the United States have included one of the following criteria: minimum age (generally aged 55 and older), physical or mental health status, and minimum sentencing and criminal risk clauses at low levels (Chiu, 2010). For details of the criterion for geriatric release, please see Maschi et al., (2016). Nevertheless, obstacles to their successful implementation have been established in the United States and other countries, even for elderly, infirm, and severely ill older adults in custody.

Consequently, rights of older persons to dignity and respect are diminished, even when dying. These hurdles include poor law design (e.g., narrow eligibility criteria), enforcement procedures (e.g., bureaucracy within the system), and legislators' "inability" to remedy the situation because of public pressure (Chiu, 2010).

A recent study (Maschi et al., 2016) analyzed the laws of humane and geriatric release in the United States using methods of content analysis. Using inductive and deductive analysis strategies, we found 47 identified federal and state laws by searching the LexisNexis legal database and using the following search terms "compassionate release," "medical parole," "geriatric prison release," "elderly and seriously ill." Therefore, of the possible 52 federal and state corrections systems—50 states, Washington D.C., and Federal Corrections—there were 47 laws for incarcerated people or their families to petition for early release based on advanced age or health. We identified six major categories of these laws: (1) physical/mental health; (2) age; (3) pathway to release decision; (4) post-release support; (5) nature of the crime (personal and criminal justice history); and (6) stage of review (Maschi et al., 2016). The federal government also has called for the reform of compassionate and geriatric release laws, given that many incarcerated people have not been released based on their current provisions (USDOJ, 2015). For instance, U.S. federal laws and policies, such as the Americans with Disability Act and Compassionate Release Laws, could be more actively used to improve conditions of confinement for older adults in prison. As of 2020, all U.S. states have such laws in place.

For parole, two policy areas that have gained considerable attention are clemency and compassionate and geriatric release laws (USDOJ, 2015). Clemency is a policy issue that has received recognition during the Obama administration and has also impacted the legal protection of older adults in prison (Shear, 2016). Clemency generally refers to an act of mercy in which a public official, such as a governor or president, has the power to reduce the harshness of the sentence or imprisonment of inmates (Shear, 2016). For example, a *New York Times* article documents Obama's "merciful" record at the federal level in which he granted 78 pardons and 153 commutations to incarcerated people. They primarily received long term sentences for drug convictions during the 1980s tough on crime era.

As illustrated in the artwork (see Figure 3), we must use multiple modalities to inform the general public of these concepts, especially the core ideas of compassion, mercy, and forgiveness, for people of all ages in order to visualize a kinder and more peaceful world.

In the Wake of the Coronavirus (COVID-19)

The aging in prison epidemic reached a critical point with the emergence and spread of the Coronavirus and even more death occurring in prisons. There is a plethora of news with reports that older adults

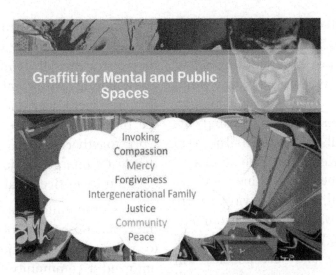

Figure 3. Graffiti for Mental and Public Spaces

and individuals with a compromised immune system are more vulnerable, especially those confined in prisons, in which proximity with each other significantly increases the risk of spreading the disease. For example, in March 2020 the American Civil Liberties Union (ACLU) sent a letter to both the United States Department of Justice (DOJ) and Bureau of Prisons (BOP) urging the facilities to protect the welfare of all incarcerated individuals, while also strongly recommending the early release of older adult offenders and those with chronic health conditions (ACLU, 2020). Furthermore, numerous states have seen jail releases for those offenders who are non-violent, medically unwell, and over the age of 60 (Prison Policy Initiative, 2020).

As health, social, cultural, and political systems seem to be in disarray, many people have lost their sense of stability. Countries and regions around the globe are currently having their people in "lockdown" and fearing for their own, their families, and communities. The current discourse in the press and social media is about spreading fear and the need to isolate each other. In other words, the concepts of isolation and incarceration become evident for those without justice involvement, yet who are prisoners of the pandemic.

As we move through the birth of the "caring justice partnership" era, we should embrace interbeing and interconnectedness as ways to bring light to the shadows of internal prisons. As exemplified by so many resilient older adults in prison, they practiced detached observation of their emotions and behaviors related to fear, shame, hatred, and violence, which allowed them to move into unconditional love, recovery, and transformation. Such a multidimensional process happens at mental, emotional, physical, social, and spiritual levels both individually and collectively.

Together, we have the ability to create a caring justice world that recognizes the divinity in one another. It starts at the individual level, by working through self-love and self-forgiveness, and then by spreading love and kindness to others. The older adults in prison taught us so much. By releasing ourselves, we will release them. The term corona also refers to the halo of the sun. Let us welcome the sunshine. Once we release the old, sick, and dying, we are making our way to embrace our humanness fully. When love is in the lead, compassionate and just policies will flow with ease, and communities will be healthier, happier, and safer.

Final Reflection

This issue of aging in prison was not created by one party alone that is aging in prison, but by us all. Together we can identify the root of the problem and solutions to why people of all ages are not safe in their communities or their prisons. Are we solving the problem by locking it out of sight in the deep recesses of the prisons of our minds? We encourage the readers to ask themselves and then others: How did we get here? Is this the situation we would want for our family members or for other people's family members with a loved one who was a victim of a crime and a perpetrator? Is this the kind of shared humanity that we want our children to inher-

it or how we wanted to be treated as grandparents? Can we envision alternative strategies to reinforce personal accountability with compassionate care for those victimized and who committed offenses? Are there other ways to work together to forge new solutions that foster intergenerational family and community justice for all?

Communities must deliberate on the costs and benefits of our approach to matters of care and justice. We recommend a community forum held in local communities that uses basic questions. How can we co-construct community that promotes health and safety for people of all ages and their communities? What are some of the strengths and challenges of getting there? What would be the ideal situation? How can we forge a path together to get there? First, visualize, then you can realize. That is the altruistic imagination and its infinite wisdom. Do it with love, then the policies and will of the people will follow. Our wise elders have never let us down. Even though many people have vilified older adults in prison, they still care and yet figured out a way to get their message out, even when it was against the odds. We encourage our readers to consider accepting the gift of life that wise older adults in prison selflessly have shared with us, and we now share with you.

"To forgive is to set a prisoner free and discover that the prisoner was you."

—Lewis B. Smedes

References

Aday, R. H. (2003). *Aging prisoners: Crisis in American corrections*. Westport, CT: Praeger.

Agnew, R. (1989). A longitudinal test of the revised strain theory. *Journal of Quantitative Criminology, 5*(4), 373-387.

American Civil Liberties Union. (2020). *ACLU Letter to DOJ and BOP on Coronavirus and the Criminal Justice System*. Retrieved April 28, 2020, from https://www.aclu.org/letter/aclu-letter-doj-and-bop-coronavirus-and-criminal-justice-system

Baillargeon, J., Williams, B. A., Mellow, J., Harzke, A. J., Hoge, S. K., Baillargeon, G., & Greifinger, R. B. (2009). Parole revocation among prison inmates with psychiatric and substance use disorders. *Psychiatric Services, 60*(11), 1516-1521.

Bartels, S. J., & Naslund, J. A. (2013). The underside of the silver tsunami—older adults and mental health care. *New England Journal of Medicine, 368*(6), 493-496.

Benfer, E., Mohapatra, S., Wiley, L., & Yearby, R. (2020). Health Justice Strategies to Combat the Pandemic: Eliminating Discrimination, Poverty, and Health Inequity During and After COVID-19. *Yale Journal of Health Policy, Law, and Ethics*, Forthcoming, Available at SSRN: https://ssrn.com/abstract=3636975

Bunce, A. (2018). Developing a Compassionate Community Compassionate Inverclyde. *International Journal of Integrated Care (IJIC), 18*(Suppl. 2), 1-2.

Chiu, T. (2010). *It's About Time: Aging Prisoners, Increasing Costs, And Geriatric Release*. Vera Institute. Retrieved from https://www.vera.org/publications/its-about-time-aging-prisoners-increasing-costs-and-geriatric-release

Codd, H. (2013). *In the shadow of prison: Families, imprisonment and criminal justice*. Willan.

Dai, W. D., & Yu, F. (2011). The correction of old prisoners: A sociological study. *China Prison Journal, 4*, 25-29.

Elder, G. H. (1974). *Children of the great depression: Social change and life experience*. Chicago, IL: University of Chicago Press.

Elder, G. H. (2003). The emergence and development of life course theory. In J. T. Mortimer & M. J. Shanahan (Eds.), *Handbook of the life course* (pp. 3–19). New York, NY: Kluwer Academic/Plenum Press Publishers.

Gilbert, P. (2009). Introducing compassion-focused therapy. *Advances in psychiatric treatment, 15*(3), 199-208.

Goetting, A. (1984). The elderly in prison: A profile. *Criminal Justice Review, 9*(2), 14-24.

Harding, D. J., Morenoff, J. D., Nguyen, A. P., & Bushway, S. D. (2017). Short-and long-term effects of imprisonment on future felony convictions and prison admissions. *Proceedings of the National Academy of Sciences, 114*(42), 11103-11108.

Human Rights Watch [HRW]. (2012). *Old Behind Bars: The Aging Prison Population in the United States.* Retrieved from https://www.hrw.org/report/ 2012/01/27/old-behind-bars/aging-prison-population-united-states

Kordowicz, M. (2019). Creating compassionate NHS organisations. *The Psychologist, 32*, 34-35.

LaLlave, J. A., & Gutheil, T. G. (2012). Expert witness and Jungian archetypes. *International Journal of Law and Psychiatry, 35*(5-6), 456-463.

Laub, J. H., & Sampson, R. J. (1993). Turning points in the life course: Why change matters to the study of crime. *Criminology, 31*(3), 301-325.

Maschi, T., & Aday, R. H. (2014). The social determinants of health and justice and the aging in prison crisis: A call for human rights action. *International Journal of Social Work, 1*(1), 15-33.

Maschi, T., & Baer, J. (2013). The heterogeneity of the world assumptions of older adults in prison: Do differing worldviews have a mental health effect?. *Traumatology, 19*(1), 65-72.

Maschi, T., & Kaye, A. (2018). *Incarcerated Older Adults.* Retrieved from https:// www.giaging.org/issues/incarcerated-older-adults/

Maschi, T., & Koskinen, L. (2015). Co-constructing community: A conceptual map for reuniting aging people in prison with their families and communities. *Traumatology, 21*(3), 208.

Maschi, T., & Leibowitz, G. (2018). Aging, stigma, and criminal justice. In W. T. Church & D. W. Springer (Eds.), *Serving the Stigmatized: Working within the Incarcerated Environment* (pp. 88-113). Oxford University Press.

Maschi, T., & Morgen, K. (2020). *Aging Behind Prison Walls: Studies in Trauma and Resilience.* New York, NY: Columbia University Press.

Maschi, T., Dennis, K. S., Gibson, S., MacMillan, T., Sternberg, S., & Hom, M. (2011). Trauma and stress among older adults in the criminal justice system: A review of the literature with implications for social work. *Journal of Gerontological Social Work, 54*(4), 390-424.

Maschi, T., Gibson, S., Zgoba, K. M., & Morgen, K. (2011). Trauma and life event stressors among young and older adult prisoners. *Journal of Correctional Health Care, 17*(2), 160-172.

Maschi, T., Kwak, J., Ko, E., & Morrissey, M. B. (2012). Forget me not: Dementia in prison. *The Gerontologist, 52*(4), 441-451.

Maschi, T., Leibowitz, G., Rees, J., & Pappacena, L. (2016). Analysis of US compassionate and geriatric release laws: Applying a human rights framework to global prison health. *Journal of Human Rights and Social Work, 1*(4), 165-174.

Maschi, T., Morgen, K., Zgoba, K., Courtney, D., & Ristow, J. (2011). Age, cumulative trauma and stressful life events, and post-traumatic stress symptoms among older adults in prison: Do subjective impressions matter?. *The Gerontologist, 51*(5), 675-686.

Maschi, T., Morrisey, M. B., & Leigey, M. (2013). The case for human agency, well-being, and community reintegration for people aging in prison: A statewide case analysis. *Journal of Correctional Health Care, 19*(3), 194-210.

Maschi, T., Viola, D., & Koskinen, L. (2015). Trauma, stress, and coping among older adults in prison: Towards a human rights and intergenerational family justice action agenda. *Traumatology, 21*(3), 188.

Maschi, T., Viola, D., & Morgen, K. (2013). Trauma and coping among older adults in prison: Linking empirical evidence to practice. *Gerontologist, 54*(5), 857-867.

Maschi, T., Viola, D., & Sun, F. (2013). The high cost of the international aging prisoner crisis: Well-being as the common denominator for action. *The Gerontologist, 53*(4), 543-554.

Maschi, T., Viola, D., Harrison, M. T., Harrison, W., Koskinen, L., & Bellusa, S. (2014). Bridging community and prison for older adults: invoking human rights and elder and intergenerational family justice. *International Journal of Prisoner Health*.

Maschi, T., Viola, D., Morgen, K., & Koskinen, L. (2015). Trauma, stress, grief, loss, and separation among older adults in prison: The protective role of coping resources on physical and mental well-being. *Journal of Crime and Justice, 38*(1), 113-136.

Merriam-Webster. (2020). Definition of Justice. In *Merriam-Webster's Collegiate*

Dictionary. Retrieved from https://www.merriam-webster.com/dictionary/justice

New York Times [Editorial]. (2017, January 3). Why Keep the Old and Sick Behind Bars? *New York Times.* Retrieved from https://www.nytimes.com/2017/01/03/opinion/why-keep-the-old-and-sick-behind-bars.html

Norris, F. H. (1992). Epidemiology of trauma: frequency and impact of different potentially traumatic events on different demographic groups. *Journal of Consulting and Clinical Psychology, 60*(3), 409-418.

Pearlin, L. I., & Skaff, M. M. (1996). Stress and the life course: A paradigmatic alliance. *The Gerontologist, 36*(2), 239-247.

Prison Policy Initiative (2020). *Responses to the COVID-19 pandemic.* Retrieved on April 27, 2020, from https://www.prisonpolicy.org/virus/virusresponse.html

Rawls, J., & and Kelly, E. I. (2003). *Justice as Fairness.* Cambridge, MA: Harvard University Press.

Sampson, R. J., & Laub, J. H. (2003). Life-course desisters? Trajectories of crime among delinquent boys followed to age 70. *Criminology, 41*(3), 555-592.

Shear, M. D. (2016, December 19). Obama's 78 Pardons and 153 Commutations Extend Record of Mercy. *New York Times.* Retrieved from https://www.nytimes.com/2016/12/19/us/politics/obama-commutations-pardons-clemency.html

Shimkus, J. (2004). The graying of America's prisons: Corrections copes with care for the aged. *Correct Care, 18*(3), 1-16.

Stojkovic, S. (2007). Elderly prisoners: A growing and forgotten group within correctional systems vulnerable to elder abuse. *Journal of Elder Abuse & Neglect, 19*(3-4), 97-117.

United Nations Office on Drugs and Crime [UNODC] (2009). *Handbook for Prisoners with Special Needs.* Vienna Austria: Author. Retrieved August 1, 2011 from https://www.unodc.org/pdf/criminal_justice/Handbook_on_Prisoners_with_Special_Needs.pdf

United States Department of Justice [USDOJ], Office of the Inspector General. (2015). The impact of an aging inmate population on the Federal Bureau of Prisons. Washington, DC: Author.

Wakefield, J. C. (1988). Psychotherapy, distributive justice, and social work: Part 1: Distributive justice as a conceptual framework for social work. *Social Service Review, 62*(2), 187-210.

West, H., & Sabol, W. (2008). Prisoners in 2007 (NCJ Publication No. 224280). Rockville, MD: U.S. Department of Justice.

Williams, B. A., Goodwin, J. S., Baillargeon, J., Ahalt, C., & Walter, L. C. (2012). Addressing the aging crisis in US criminal justice health care. *Journal of the American Geriatrics Society, 60*(6), 1150-1156.

Perspectives on Aging-Related Preparation

Silvia Sörensen, PhD*

Rachel L. Missell, MS

Alexander Eustice-Corwin, MA

Dorine A. Otieno, MS, MPH

*Margaret Warner Graduate School for Education
and Human Development, University of Rochester*

*Corresponding Author: Silvia Sörensen, PhD, Associate Professor, Counseling and
Human Development, Warner School of Education and Human Development:
ssorensen@warner.rochester.edu

ABSTRACT

When older adults face age-related life challenges, anticipating
what to expect and how to access potential coping strategies can
both prevent and provide the possibility of easier recovery from
crises. Aging-Related Preparation (ARP) is defined as the continuum of thoughts and activities about how to age well, often beginning with the awareness of age-related changes, or the anticipation
of retirement, and concluding with specifying end-of-life wishes.
In the current paper, we introduce the concept of ARP and related
formulations regarding plans for aging well, describe both predictors and outcomes of ARP for several the domains of ARP, and
consider the elements of ARP within the context of existing social
policy. We conclude that ARP is determined by a variety of influences both intrinsic to the older person (e.g., personality, cognitive
ability, beliefs about planning, problem-solving skills), linked to social class and education, as well as dependent on family structures,
access to and knowledge of options, services, and local community
resources, and social policy. We further provide evidence that ARP
has positive effects in the domain of pre-retirement planning (for
retirement adjustment), of preparation for future care (for emotional well-being), and of ACP (for a good death). However, other
domains of ARP, including planning for leisure, housing, and social planning are under-researched. Finally, we discuss policy implications of the existing research.

Keywords: Age-related preparation, Retirement planning, Preparation for future care, Proactive Coping, Long-term care

doi: 10.18278/jep.1.2.7

Perspectivas sobre la preparación relacionada con el envejecimiento

Resumen

Cuando los adultos mayores enfrentan desafíos de la vida relacionados con la edad, anticipar qué esperar y cómo acceder a posibles estrategias de afrontamiento puede prevenir y brindar la posibilidad de una recuperación más fácil de las crisis. La preparación relacionada con el envejecimiento (ARP) se define como el continuo de pensamientos y actividades sobre cómo envejecer bien, a menudo comenzando con la conciencia de los cambios relacionados con la edad o la anticipación de la jubilación, y concluyendo con la especificación de los deseos del final de la vida. En el artículo actual, presentamos el concepto de ARP y formulaciones relacionadas con respecto a los planes para envejecer bien, describimos tanto los predictores como los resultados de ARP para varios dominios de ARP y consideramos los elementos de ARP dentro del contexto de la política social existente. Concluimos que el ARP está determinado por una variedad de influencias tanto intrínsecas a la persona mayor (p. Ej., Personalidad, capacidad cognitiva, creencias sobre la planificación, habilidades para la resolución de problemas), vinculadas a la clase social y la educación, así como dependientes de las estructuras familiares. acceso y conocimiento de opciones, servicios y recursos de la comunidad local, y política social. Además, proporcionamos evidencia de que ARP tiene efectos positivos en el dominio de la planificación previa a la jubilación (para el ajuste de la jubilación), de la preparación para la atención futura (para el bienestar emocional) y de la ACP (para una buena muerte). Sin embargo, se están investigando otros dominios de ARP, incluida la planificación del ocio, la vivienda y la planificación social. Finalmente, discutimos las implicaciones políticas de la investigación existente.

Palabras clave: Preparación relacionada con la edad, planificación de la jubilación, preparación para la atención futura, afrontamiento proactivo, atención a largo plazo

关于老龄化相关准备的视角

摘要

当老年人面临老龄化相关的生活挑战时，预期未来规划以及如何获取可能的应对策略能防止危机并提供从危机中快速恢复的机会。老龄化相关准备（ARP）被定义为关于如何健康老去的想法和活动的连续体，经常以意识到老龄化相关变化、或预期退休开始，以确定遗愿结束。本文中，我们引入了ARP概念和有关健康老去规划的相关定义，描述了几个ARP领域中ARP的预测物和结果，衡量了现有社会政策背景下ARP的各要素。我们的结论认为，ARP由一系列影响因素决定，这些影响因素不仅是老年人所固有的（例如性格、认知能力、关于规划的信念、问题解决技能），与社会阶层和教育相联系，并且取决于家庭结构、对选择、服务和地方社区资源的获取及理解、以及社会政策。我们进一步提供证据证明，ARP在退休前规划（用于退休调整）、未来护理准备（用于情感福祉）、ACP（用于善终）这三个领域中具有积极效果。不过，其他ARP领域，包括娱乐规划、住房和社会规划，还有待研究。最后，我们探讨了现有研究的政策意义。

关键词：老龄化相关准备，退休规划，未来护理准备，主动应对（Proactive Coping），长期护理

Perspectives on Aging-Related Preparation

Planning for the future is considered a common activity among young adults seeking to exert agency over their own development (Lerner & Busch-Rossnagel, 1981). Among older adults, however, future preparation is much less the norm (Freund et al., 2009). When older adults face age-related life challenges, being able to imagine what to expect and how to access potential coping strategies is a "mental dress rehearsal" (Evans et al., 1985, p. 369). Whether older adults can achieve positive developmental outcomes and maintain well-being as they age may depend in part on the extent to which they have engaged in preparation activities or developmental regulation. Aging-Related Preparation (ARP) is defined as the continuum of thoughts and activities about how to age well, often beginning with the awareness of age-related changes, or the anticipation of retirement and concluding with specifying end-of-life wishes. Early goals and plans revolve around leisure, social relationships, and housing transitions; later plans focus on preparation for health challenges, the loss of loved ones, and managing situations in which autonomous decisions may be compromised by dementia or other severe illness (Baltes & Smith, 2003; Lang, Baltes & Wagner, 2007; Sörensen et al., 2012). Vital to effective aging-related preparation is recognizing the risks for aging-related losses and identifying potential resources to managing those challenges. As Lang and Rupprecht (2019) note "aging may also involve the need to accept some kind of vulnerability" (p. 2).

Demographics, labor markets, and policy shifts have contributed to an increase in the importance of individual and family-based ARP. In response to the increasing proportion of older adults in the population, declining birthrates, the baby boom cohorts retiring, and the resulting decrease in number of working adults per older person in most industrialized countries (e.g., Social Security Administration, 2020; Vincent & Velkoff, 2010; Bogetic et al., 2015), more governments expect their citizens to be individually responsible for preparing for old age, rather than relying primarily on government services with regard to financial retirement planning, housing, and receiving care (Preston et al., 2019; Soichit, & Khophai, 2017; Niu et al., 2020).

The purpose of the current paper is to explain the process and domains of Aging-Related Preparation and to discuss how the findings in this area of study are relevant to aging policy. While we aim to address the primary

issues in this field, this review is not comprehensive. To orient the reader, we briefly review the concept of ARP and the theoretical basis for ARP; then we summarize the current findings regarding the nature of, reported frequency, predictors, and outcomes of ARP; finally, we the explore the policy implications of these findings, in view of social policy and intervention. Given our concern with policy relevance, we focus, with some exceptions, on findings from the U.S. and from the last 10-15 years, during which the baby boomers have begun to retire.

The Concept of Aging-Related Preparation

Our concept of Aging-Related Preparation (ARP) encompasses several related preparation activities: *pre-retirement planning* (e.g., Baltes & Rudolph, 2012; Donaldson et al., 2010; Freund et al., 2009; Löckenhoff, 2012), *preparation for future care* (e.g., Pinquart et al., 2017; Sörensen & Pinquart, 2000a), *housing decisions* (Adams & Rau, 2011; Oswald et al., 2006), and *advance care planning* (e.g., Detering et al., 2010; Hines, 2001; Dixon et al., 2018). Across these contexts, we consider planning and preparation as life-span processes (Freund et al., 2009; Löckenhoff, 2012) in a multi-domain environment (Kornadt & Rothermund, 2014). A related concept is *preparation for age-related changes*, which defines multiple domains of preparation for old age (Kornadt et al., 2020). ARP is distinguished from this literature by its focus on *processes,* as informed by the psychology of everyday cognitive planning (e.g., Berg et al., 1997; Craik & Byalistok, 2006; Das et al., 1996; Friedman & Scholnick, 2014; Scholnick & Friedman, 1993; Hayes-Roth & Hayes-Roth, 1979; Rebok, 1989). Combining the literature on cognitive planning and preparation for future care (Sörensen et al., 2011), ARP processes include, for example, awareness of the need for aging-related preparation (due, perhaps, to a loss of mobility), gathering information about future threats and options (e.g., difficulty with stairs necessitating single-level house or assisted living), making decisions about goals and preferences (e.g., wanting to maximize privacy), and enacting preliminary steps (e.g., seeking a new house). In addition, the study of ARP is informed by the literature on goal setting.

Goal Setting. Establishing goal states toward which to strive can organize an individual's active engagement in their own development. Goal setting is considered a critical element of successful aging and better health (Fisher & Specht, 1999; Fooken, 1982) or a "good old age" (Street & Desai, 2011). Mental representations of successful aging (Rowe & Kahn, 1997) can be described as *possible selves* (Cross & Markus, 1991; Markus & Nurius, 1986), *developmental tasks* (Hutteman et al., 2014), *personal life tasks* (Cantor et al., 1991), *life goals* (Nurmi, 1992), *personal goals* (Brunstein, Schultheiss & Maier, 1999; Riediger, Freund & Baltes, 2005), *personal projects* (Little, Salmela-Aro & Phillips, 2017), *personal strivings* (Emmons, 1989; 1999), and *personal life investment* (Schindler & Staudinger, 2008).

Older adults report different goals than younger adults (Strough et al., 1996), with older adults' goals centering around health and health maintenance, retirement adjustment, sleep, chores, community, recreation, and spirituality (Chen et al., 2012), maintenance/loss prevention, present-day experiences and emotions, generativity, and social selection (Penningroth & Scott, 2012), and independent living (G. Carstensen et al., 2019). Kornadt et al. (2020) outline eleven domains of preparation for age-related changes covering both the "Third age" (ca. ages 60-80) when retirement, continued activity, generativity, and health maintenance are salient (Laslett, 1989), and the "Fourth age" of increasing frailty and loss of functioning associated with advanced old age (Baltes & Smith, 2003; Gilleard & Higgs, 2011). Below, goal setting is discussed as a component of the four most researched domains of ARP (pre-retirement planning, preparation for future care, housing decisions, and advance care planning).

Theoretical Considerations. Aging-related Preparation is informed by several theoretical approaches, including theories of proactive coping (Aspinwall & Taylor, 1997), the model of *Selection, Optimization, and Compensation* (Baltes & Baltes, 1990), and theories of life-span control (Heckhausen & Schulz, 1995). Regarding proactive coping, ARP is recognized as a way to manage future stressors either by *preventing* some of them or *coping* with them more effectively (Berg et al., 1997) by developing *potential responses* to physical and cognitive health stressors (Aspinwall, 2005). Selection, Optimization, and Compensation suggests specific actions that assist with adjustment to aging-related changes, such as the *selection* of valued activities (e.g., ones that are safer), *optimization* of goals (e.g., social, activity, and independence goals by moving to a less demanding but more social environment, like assisted living; see, e.g., Perry & Thiels, 2016), and *compensation* for age-related losses (e.g., through the use of assistive devices; see Freedman et al., 2017). Life-span control theories (Heckhausen & Schulz, 1995) suggest that the use of primary control strategies, such as seeking out new activities and friends and engaging in preventive action, and secondary control strategies, such as regulating the emotions resulting from the prospect of future loss and the actual experienced losses (Löckenhoff, 2012) through flexible goal adjustment (Brandtstädter, 2009; Brandtstädter & Rothermund, 2003). Finally, the notion that making plans helps bridge the intention–behavior gap for older adults (Reuter et al., 2010) presents a potential *mechanism* for the benefit of ARP.

Notably, the conceptualization of ARP is also consistent with the theory of preventive and corrective proactivity (Kahana et al., 2012). Similar to SOC and life-span theories of control, this conceptualization suggests that older adults can perceive threats to future goal states, such as to their future emotional well-being, and select environments, behaviors, and responses, thus attempting to control their quality of life (to a certain extent) in advance of predictable age-related losses. Howev-

er, the motivation for ARP is likely influenced by the perceived control over these events and beliefs about the time frame within which these threats are likely to occur (Ouwehand et al., 2007) as well as the *type* of event. For example, preparation for unexpected events, such as falls and fractures or financial setbacks due to stock market crashes, is considerably less likely than planning for age-related changes that are either normative or easily anticipated, such as loss of physical strength or the need for stronger visual aids.

In sum, whereas the ARP literature incorporates a sociological understanding of societal and contextual influences, especially with regard to demographics, policy change, and pre-retirement planning, it is at its core an application of life-span developmental approaches to self-management in late life for retirement, preparation for managing gains and losses of aging, living with chronic illness (Barlow et al., 2016; Greenglass et al., 2006; Heckhausen et al., 2013), future health care anticipation and determining preferences, housing decisions, as well as dying with dignity (for which there appears to be no current theorizing). Thus, while we acknowledge the role that the sociological understanding, especially the understanding of cross-cultural and policy research has played in the development of the ARP literature, our theoretical emphasis relies more explicitly on life-span developmental approaches to aging and ARP.

Findings Regarding ARP

Four topics dominate the empirical literature in ARP. These include the frequency of ARP in different populations and at what level of concreteness or extent it typically occurs; the predisposing and facilitating factors, as well as the barriers to ARP among older adults; the evidence for the usefulness of ARP for health and well-being outcomes; and attempts to increase aging-related preparation among older populations.

How Much Do People Prepare?

The extent to which older adults report preparation in different domains varies by samples and measurement tools, and how questions are asked. Also, the extent and concreteness of preparation does not speak to the quality or realism of plans.

Retirement Planning

Research on pre-retirement planning has emphasized that age-normed transitions constitute turning points (Stenholm & Vahtera, 2017) affecting the individual's *financial stability* (e.g., Hershey & Mowen, 2000), necessitating *psychological adjustment* to changes in work demands and social opportunities (e.g., Wang & Shi, 2014), and requiring *preparation* for the financial and psychological effects of retirement-related transitions (e.g., Adams & Rau, 2011; Earl & Archibald, 2014; Gonzales & Nowell, 2017; Löckenhoff, 2012; Street & Desai, 2011; Wang & Shi, 2014). Critiques of this literature suggest that the predominantly male-centered framing

of retirement as an abrupt change is less relevant to women (Loretto & Vickerstaff, 2013) and Baby Boomers (e.g., Kojola & Moen, 2016) who are redefining retirement as a more gradual process with periods of non-work, part-time work, and return to work. A historical focus on financial aspects of retirement in the research (e.g., Appleton, 1900; Buck, 1926; Meriam, 1918; Hershey & Mowen, 2000) is now counterbalanced by studies investigating multiple domains of retirement planning including psychological (career and employment decisions, leisure/recreation), financial (income, employment, estate planning), psychosocial (social and interpersonal), and health-related preparation (Hershey et al., 2001; Yeung, 2013).

Active retirement planning that incorporates non-financial plans into retirement preparation, however, is rarely performed by American workers; fewer than 1/4 engage in planning for *where* they would retire or whether they would continue employment during retirement (Turner et al., 1994). Ferraro (1990) reports that about 40-60% of a nationally representative sample of 3,464 U.S. pre-retirees aged 18-67 who were surveyed in 1974 engaged in each of seven preparation activities.[1] More recently, only 12% of workers aged 51 to 61 report that they do not know or have not thought about their retirement timeframe, and about 43% report having "no plans" about the *form* of their retirement (Ekerdt et al., 2001). Thus, retirement preparation beyond finances is quite limited.

Although pre-retirees report seeking information about retirement from other retirees, coworkers, company officials, Social Security personnel, general reading, and the media (Evans et al., 1985), most retirement planning still focuses on financial planning. However, rates vary widely across studies (Ameriks et al., 2003; Bucher-Koenen & Lusardi, 2011) and many people report rather cursory plans. For example, only 29% of TIAA-CREF participants "agreed" or "strongly agreed" to have spent "a great deal of time" developing a financial plan (Ameriks et al., 2002). Results from the Retirement Confidence Survey suggest 37% of American workers have given *little or no thought* to their retirement and that only about one-third report having calculated their financial needs for a comfortable retirement (Dickemper & Yakoboski, 1997). Only about a quarter of baby boomers (currently ranging from age 56 to 74) are financially prepared for later life—60 percent will not be able to maintain their current lifestyle without continued employment, and 60 percent suffer from chronic health problems; one quarter have a current average income of only $15,000 (Court et al., 2007).

Preparation for Future Care (PFC)

Almost 70% of adults over 65 will require some type of long-term care services during their lifetime (U.S. Department of Health and Human Services, 2017), but only 37% believe that they will need these services (AARP Public Policy Institute, 2007). Most elders underestimate their potential future needs for assistance and report rarely or never thinking about these

needs (Walz & Mitchell, 2007). This evinces a need on the part of aging individuals to engage in more substantive Preparation for Future Care (PFC), defined as thoughts and activities focused on how to obtain assistance with daily tasks or personal care, as well as enact housing adjustments that allow the individual to age well. Informed by models of cognitive processes in everyday planning situations (e.g., Berg et al., 1997; Craik & Byalistok, 2006; Scholnick & Friedman, 1993; Hayes-Roth & Hayes-Roth, 1979; Rebok, 1989), PFC is described as a series of steps, from a general awareness of the need to plan, to enacting and evaluating concrete plans for specific care options. Drawing on qualitative, life-history data from a study of 51 mid-life and older Canadians, Denton and colleagues (2004) propose that *anticipating risk* of gains and losses, as well as recognizing the need to manage that risk, and understanding the life conditions that contribute to risk, should result in "reflexive planning." Sörensen et al. (2011), discussing preparation for late-life transitions, suggest that awareness of risk must be followed by *information-seeking* about the present situation, potential future threats, as well as available options (see also Ouwehand et al., 2007), as well as determining future goal states or *preferences, comparing* various options for reaching these goals, *deciding* on specific steps to take, and following up with steps that ensure access to those options (e.g., putting one's name on a waiting list). This process is depicted in Figure 1. Once needs emerge, the authors suggest that *implementing* these plans will be easier—and better—than turning to ad hoc solutions, and *evalu-* *ating plan effectiveness* will allow their calibration (Sörensen et al., 2011).

Figure 1.Preparation for Future Care as Process

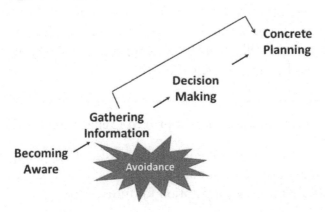

Both early and more recent studies of PFC note a distinct lack of concern about future illness and care among older adults. In 1965, Heyman and Jeffers (1965) reported that that 50% of older adults in North Carolina said they were **not** concerned about a future long-term illness, and only 16% expressed that they were "very concerned" (cf. Kulys & Tobin, 1980, who report 43% anticipate future care need). Thirty years later, 70% of older women in three-generation families said they had *thought about* what to do if they needed help with personal care and 63% had talked to others about it, but only 9% reported having made *concrete* plans (Sörensen & Zarit, 1996). Although older Americans worry more about paying for long-term care than paying for retirement, 48% of have done little or no long-term care preparation (National Council on Aging and John Hancock Mutual Life Insurance Company, 1999). In an AARP survey, about half of informal caregivers to adults of all ages say their care recipi-

ent has made *no plans* for future care or they are unsure if plans exist, 40% if the care recipient is a spouse. If the care recipient is over 50 or has dementia, the likelihood of preparation increases. Only 40% of the caregivers have plans for their *own* care (AARP Public Policy Institute & National Alliance for Caregiving, 2015). It is also worrisome that just 9% of seniors have talked with a financial professional about long term care (Age Wave & Harris Interactive, 2010). Baby boomers, although they have a higher rate of chronic illnesses than the previous generations (Soldo et al., 2006), are also not likely to have long-term care plans; 2/3 are concerned about their health in retirement and 71 percent about health care costs (Court et al., 2007).

The lack of preparation for care becomes even more apparent when broken down by its concreteness: Among women 64 and older, about one third rely primarily on others (individuals or organizations) to plan their care (Girling & Morgan, 2014), whereas 34%

engage in "autonomous planning," and the rest report awareness of preferences, but have taken no action, avoid planning altogether, or engage in unrealistic wishful thinking, staying mostly disengaged from care preparation. Similarly, 30%-52% of community dwelling older adults report general plans for their future needs with no specific notion of how to implement these preferences, but only 1% to 15% report having *concrete* plans for their care (Black et al., 2008; Sörensen & Pinquart, 2001b); 55% state that they have no plans at all for future care (Sörensen & Pinquart, 2001b).

BOX 1. Policy Recommendations for Improved Preparation for Care:

- The provision of a basic income for all caregivers of the young, disabled or old at home, most of whom are women unable to take up paid employment, would increase preparation for future care.

- Information on services for elder care must be more easily accessible both by website and in brochures available at medical centers, dementia care clinics, senior centers, local community and recreation centers, and grocery stores. Older adults and their families need easy access to information.

- Policies requiring the training and perhaps registration of formal caregivers are needed to ensure the steady availability of well-trained care providers, whose schedules are organized in communication with consumers, thus enabling long-term care planning around family and work schedules.

Housing decisions often emerge once older adults are already retired. They may include care considerations, but this is not always the case. The majority (78%) of middle-aged and older adults surveyed by the AARP in 2014 preferred to "age in place" (Barrett, 2014), particularly rural elders (e.g., Carver et al., 2018). Due to advances in telemedicine, health monitoring systems, home dialysis, and other in-home aging and medical services, it is possible to age in place, but aging in place requires careful planning to include home modifications, access to medical care and social contact, home upkeep, and contingency plans (Erickson et al., 2006).

In the housing domain goals and plans are often not aligned. Despite the fact that 49% of workers and retirees in upstate New York expect to stay in their own homes without modifications (Robison & Moen, 2000), only a small percentage of these persons have an entrance without steps, a walk-in shower, or the ability to live on one floor; repair and maintenance tasks are often deferred (Begley & Lambie-Hanson, 2015;

Kelly, 2014), both because of financial reasons and the inability to coordinate the work. Aging in place is threatened by increases in property taxes and utility costs, changes in family composition, and diminished health, whereas greater home equity, financial resources, and stronger community ties contribute to a higher likelihood of aging in place (Sabia, 2008). Also, many home modifications are not possible for renters to implement. Thus, renters are four times more likely to move in a two-year period than homeowners who hold mortgages (Robison & Moen, 2000) and thus often find it difficult to plan for aging in place.

Plans for moving are equally inadequate. In a qualitative study of older adults in the UK who had recently moved to "age-appropriate" housing, most had moved on an ad hoc basis in response to illness rather than planning housing transitions (Tulle-Winton,

1999). Whereas 20% of older Australians in their late 70s expect to move in the next ten years, most do not have firm plans (Byles et al., 2018). However, comparing Baby Boomers to older generations suggests that, unlike their plans for finances and care, Boomers' plans for housing are somewhat more realistic, including moves to apartments, retirement communities or assisted living, or living with an adult child (Robison et al., 2014). What stands out, in this literature, is that despite the desire to "age in place," many older adults are unable or unwilling to do critical decision making until they have limited choice or are unable to make a good decision. Without housing preparation, mismatches between the home and the capabilities of its older residents, especially for adults over age 85 (Levitt, 2013), can quickly lead to an unexpected or undesired relocation to a nursing home.

BOX 2. Policy Recommendations for Improved Housing Preparation:

- A holistic approach to housing policy is needed that takes into account that for older adults housing is not only a care location, or a dwelling place, but also a place to get one's social, leisure, mental and physical needs met, and to feel "at home" (Roy et al., 2018).

- Provide or expand programs that support home modification to give older persons the ability to age in place (Pynoos, 2018).

- Increase public transportation for older adults to have access to shopping, social and medical amenities, families and friends, when driving is not an option.

- Increase the supply of subsidized supportive housing by building new complexes and adding services to those that already exist. Apply the principles of universal design to meet the needs of residents of all ages, to avoid unwanted age segregation (Pynoos, 2018).

- The needs of older women should be researched more thoroughly, as those widowed or newly single may require different housing options.

- Adjust building and zoning codes for a greater range of housing options, including shared housing, co-housing, and construction-added dwelling units (Pynoos, 2018).

- Provide or expand in-home health and assistance services and their coverage through Medicare so that older adults are not forced to leave their homes.

- In congregate housing for frail older adults, not only resident safety, but also the sense of meaning older adults draw from their homes need to be taking into consideration, allowing older adults to plan for and adapt to their new dwellings and rebuild their feeling of being-at-home (Roy et al., 2018).

- Achieve better coordination of housing, health, and social service programs (Pynoos, 2018).

Advance Care Planning

The lack of attention to proactively gathering information and making decisions about care preferences (Carrese et al., 2002; Sörensen & Pinquart, 2001) has raised concerns about how older adults' care needs and preferences will be met (Court et al., 2007; Moses, 2011). Similar concerns about ACP, including designation of a health care proxy, completion of a living will, and, in some states, the completion of a Physician's Orders for Life Sustaining Treatment forms, or a "Do Not Resuscitate" order (DNR) has been expressed in the last two decades (Detering et al., 2019).

Empirical research on Advance Care Planning (ACP) emerged after passage of the Patient Self-determination Act of 1990, when clinicians observed that advance directives are mandated and advocated, but poorly understood. About one-quarter of Americans of all ages have completed an advance care planning document (Rao et al., 2014). In a review of 148 studies, ACP rates among elders were just 26.7% (averaged across all the studies, Yadav et al., 2017), but 78% for people with multiple chronic illnesses. Particularly for critically ill patients and older adults with dementia, communicating end-of-life preferences is important, as they can lose their ability to communicate. Because data on ACP discussions or advance directives completion rates are not standardized, reports of ACP rates are highly variable and difficult to interpret.

Older adults in institutional settings, and frail homebound older adults or those enrolled in special programs related to advanced care needs, are most likely to have completed some type of advanced directives (Gerst & Burr, 2008). In a nationwide survey of over 3,700 nursing home residents in 1996, about 58% had at least one type of advance care document (Degenholtz et al., 2002), but rates among adult day center attendees are 41% (Lendon et al., 2020). Among frail older adults, 66% to 81% of Caucasian and African Americans, but only 39.1% of Hispanics (Black et al., 2008; Eleazar et al., 1996; Golden et al., 2009) report at least one ACP document. Ethnic minorities report informal talks about their end-of life wishes (60%), but fewer (30%) have a durable power of attorney for health care, or living will (26.5%; Hong & Kim, 2020).

In sum, while retirement planning, preparation for future care needs, and housing preparation are not well-established among the older adult population, advance care planning is increasingly common, especially in the form of informal conversations. How much aging-related preparation occurs in other domains, such as, leisure planning, planning for maintenance of social ties, has rarely been reported. However, Baby Boomers appear at higher risk than older generations for not having engaged in much ARP (regarding health, financial resources) and many are at risk for ending up alone in old age. Boomers appear to have high levels of, perhaps unrealistic, optimism, believing that they can control their own destiny and survive anything life throws at them (78%; Court et al., 2007), whereas the very old have more accurate perceptions of their vulnerability (Kotter-Grühn et al., 2010).

Facilitating and Inhibiting Factors for Aging-Related Preparation

As we have seen, the intention to age well does not guarantee the enactment of retirement plans or care preparations. In order to translate intention into action, one needs sufficient internal and external resources. Due to cognitive deficits, lack of education, or limited problem-solving skills, older adults may lack the skills or resources needed to make age-related preparations. Lack of available aging services in their region, lack of caregivers who can assist them, no acceptable residential care, or simply limited financial means are all considerable barriers. Barriers and facilitators to ARP may occur at multiple levels including intra-individual/ psychological, family and work, community and neighborhood, wage and health care policy, inequitable structure, national policy, sociocultural, as well as historical change-levels. The interactions between levels also play a role in ARP. Which of these dominates has not been determined in the literature to date.

Psychological Factors in Aging-Related Preparation

At the Intra-individual level, personal resources, such as physical health, cognitive functioning and reserves, problem-solving skills, emotional regulation, physical health, and personal beliefs about control and planning may play a role in the initiation and shaping of ARP.

Age-related Changes in Cognitive Processing and Functioning. Individual-level age-related changes affect how much older adults engage in behaviors that promote or protect health; these include increased need for assistance with activities of daily living, and diminished health status, as well as changes in information processing and social cognition. To initiate ARP in the health care arena, a level of awareness of the risks for disease-related disability is needed (Apouye, 2018; Slovic et al., 2004), but seriously considering one's chance of frailty or dependence is often unpleasant and thus avoided (Pinquart & Sörensen, 2002; Sörensen & Pinquart, 2000b). Indeed, older adults are more likely than the young to focus on affective information in the context of decisions (Finucane, 2008), especially positive (versus negative) information (Löckenhoff & L.L. Carstensen, 2007; Mather & L.L. Carstensen, 2005), thus blocking out potential negatively valenced options for care. In addition, they tend to overestimate the negative effects on their well-being of options they *don't* like (e.g., moving to age-friendly housing) without considering potential benefits, whereas they recollect primarily positive information about the ones they prefer. These age-related changes serve to optimize immediate emotional experience and well-being (L.L. Carstensen et al., 2003), but may be somewhat deleterious to longer-term outcomes.

In addition to changes in processing positive and negative information, ARP is likely affected by both normal and pathological neuroanatomical changes that occur with aging. Changes in cortical and subcortical regions of the brain (Owen et al.,1997; Unterrainer & Owen, 2006) may affect individuals' ability make good decisions and plan a course of action (Elliott, 2003; Sanders & Schmitter-Edgecombe, 2012) or maintain an optimal level of problem-solving skill. Individuals with better problem-solving skills are more likely able to address current and potential future care problems effectively (Point Du Jour & Sörensen, 2009). Rational problem-solving styles enhance engagement in PFC, whereas dependent and avoidant decision styles inhibit it (Sörensen & Pinquart, 2001b). Decision-making competence affects the quality of retirement planning (Parker et al., 2012).

Cognitive barriers to ARP also include lack of insight into its usefulness (Blackwood et al., 2019) and about the available options for care (Delgadillo et al., 2004). Knowledge of services and health literacy are often enhanced by higher educational achievement, thus disadvantaging individuals with lower education are often lacking in requirements for the ARP process. In addition, older adults are often ill-informed about how formal long-term care is paid for, believing that having paid into Medicare and Social Security qualifies them for long-term care services.

Salience of Health Threat. Whereas age-related changes in information-seeking and decision making may thwart effective ARP, the salience of potential health threats increases plans for health and care (Ouwehand et al., 2008a), although findings are somewhat inconsistent. For example, age is related to *more* preparation for housing decisions, finances, emergencies, and health among German respondents (Kornadt & Rothermund, 2014), whereas need for ADL assistance and poor self-rated health is related to *less* concrete planning for future health needs among older adults in Florida (Black et al., 2008); but poor health predicts *more* concrete planning among seniors in Utah and Eastern Germany (Sörensen & Pinquart, 2000c). Contradictions in the literature describing the relationship of age and PFC may be attributable to these counteracting forces.

In sum, although "normal" aging does not necessarily prompt more ARP, specific triggers do. Some studies find that among individuals with specific disabilities, such as Multiple Sclerosis, functional losses are mourned and addressed more readily, making room for action to organize supports, and to contemplate future needs (Finalyson & Van Denend, 2003). In the context of policy, these findings suggest that neither scare tactics, nor a focus on future disease and disability are likely to motivate aging-related preparation. Rather, learning to concretize vague goals for a "good" old age, and more accessible information about housing and care options may spark more consideration of that information for oneself.

Mastery and Self-efficacy. Mastery, or the degree to which one feels one has a sense of control over what occurs in one's life, is an important factor in whether older adults engage in ARP. For example, after controlling for the effects of demographics and health, both a higher personal sense of mastery and more favorable retirement conditions significantly influenced adjustment to retirement post-retirement planning among Australian middle-aged and older adults (Donaldson et al., 2010).

Mastery and Self-efficacy may also play a role in the tendency of older adults to neglect spelling out plans or action steps (e.g., commitment to, initiation of, and persistence in goal pursuit) to achieve their goals as compared to younger adults (e.g., Brandtstätter, et al., 2001; G. Carstensen et al., 2019; Schnitzspahn & Kliegel, 2009; Zanjari et al., 2016). The lack of translation of goals into action steps raises the question whether specific processes operating in ARP vary across life domains and are differentially facilitated by factors internal (e.g., attitudes, knowledge, skills, personality) and external (e.g., family, community, culture) to the individual, or whether it matters whether the goals are oriented more toward goal attainment (approach) or avoidance of losses (Marsiske et al., 1995). Self-efficacy also enables older adults to respond to stress with more effective strategies for problem-solving (Li & Yang, 2009). Older adults with low self-efficacy for planning and problem-solving may find that it is not worthwhile to expend their energy making decisions. They may prefer that trusted family members plan for them (Funk, 2004; Girling & Morgan, 2014).

Attitudes and Beliefs. Engagement in ARP is highly dependent on attitudes. Negative and ambivalent attitudes toward retirement are associated with less retirement preparation and failure to seek information about retirement (Eckerdt et al., 2001; Kim & Moen, 2001; Chan et al., 2020). With regard to PFC, attitudes include the belief that care planning is useful, which predicts the likelihood of enacting specific ARP behaviors, such as Gathering Information and Concrete Planning (Sörensen & Pinquart, 2001b). Of course, attitudes can also be a function of underlying external factors, such as community norms. These include beliefs about the outcomes of planning in general. Individuals who reach adulthood in contexts that leave little freedom to plan, such as older adults in former East Germany, are less likely to believe that planning for care is useful (Pinquart & Sörensen, 2002; Sörensen & Pinquart, 2000b). Having a nonaccepting attitude toward planning is also related to reduced likelihood of engaging in both PFC (Sörensen & Pinquart, 2000a) and ACP (Black et al., 2008). Mak and Sörensen (2012), in a longitudinal study of first-degree relatives of Alzheimer's patients in the United States, show that a belief in the usefulness of planning robustly predicts lower baseline Avoidance and more Gathering Information as well as an increase in Decision Making and Concrete Planning over a 6.5-year period.

Religious beliefs may affect older adults' likelihood to engage in Aging-Related Preparation, but findings are inconsistent. Being Catholic is relat-ed to a 52% lower likelihood of engaging in PFC or ACP in one study (Black et al., 2008), but higher in another (for both Catholic and Jewish elders; Ejaz, 2000), with no relation in a third (Cohen-Mansfield et al.,1992). The sense that "God will take care of me" appears in several qualitative studies as a barrier to both PFC and ACP (Sörensen & Pinquart, 2000b; Girling & Morgan, 2014). Non-religious adults are more likely than religious ones to complete advance directives (Rurup et al., 2006).

Future time perspective has emerged as another attitudinal variable. A qualitative study by Denton et al. (2004) shows that preparation for late life is associated with a forward-looking future-time perspective. Having a limited time perspective is linked to more preparation in one study (Fowler & Fisher, 2009), but, in others, expected longevity is related to more preparation for finances, housing, and health (Apouye, 2018; Kornadt & Rothermund, 2015) as well as general retirement preparation (Jacobs-Lawson & Hershey, 2005). Participants who report clearer goal expectations for their future prepare more concretely for fitness, social relations, and leisure activities, whereas shorter subjective remaining lifetime is related to more preparation for housing, finances, emergencies, and health care four years later (Kornadt et al., 2018). Also, future orientation is associated with proactive coping for health, social relationships and personal finance in mid and late life (Ouwehand et al., 2008a). Planful attitudes and belief in continuity may enhance older adults' ability to foster their own planning competency, such as sequencing their activities along a timeline spanning from the current situation to a desired future state (Fretz et al., 1989; Sterns et al., 2005).

From a policy perspective, a shift toward a forward-looking time perspective requires shifts both at the individual and the societal level. ARP is likely to be attempted by more people when they are able to (1) imagine positive aging, (2) access information about resources, (3) receive help with problem-solving skills, and (4) know they can access affordable quality care regardless of income or assets. Current policies advantage those who are already able to access these supports.

Personality, Future Time Perspective, and Mental Health. A wealth of literature attests to the fact that retirement planning is affected by psychological factors, including personality indicators such as conscientiousness (Hershey & Mowen, 2000), emotional stability (Blekesaune & Skirbekk, 2012; Juson & Klat, 2013), risk tolerance or aversion (Dohmen et al., 2011; Grable & Lytoon, 2003), and future time perspective (Bernheim et al., 1997). Other factors noted in the literature regarding financial decision making are future expectations (Lusardi, 1999), clearly formulated financial goals (Neukam & Hershey, 2003; Stawski et al., 2007), current asset allocation (Vora & McGinnis, 2000), attitudes related to the financial planning process (Jacobs-Lawson & Hershey, 2005), and emotion regulation regarding aging-related fears, worries, or losses (Glass & Kilpatrick, 1998; Löckenhoff, 2012; Neukam & Hershey, 2003).

Psychological factors play a role in PFC and ACP as well. Personality traits, such as Openness to new experience, and Agreeableness are positively associated with greater Awareness of care needs, as is Neuroticism; Gathering Information and less Avoidance are also linked to greater Openness (Sörensen et al., 2008). Regarding end-of life planning, higher levels of conscientiousness and openness predict discussions of end-of-life plans, whereas higher levels of conscientiousness and agreeableness are linked to a greater likelihood of formal advance care planning (Ha & Pai, 2012). Trait-level optimism and hope have also been investigated with regard to future care plans. Whereas higher levels of hope are associated with more concrete planning and decision-making about future care (Southerland et al., 2016), greater optimism predicts gathering information and concrete planning (Sörensen et al., 2014). Lower hopefulness is associated with greater *awareness* of future care needs, however.

Depression is independently associated with PFC, particularly gathering information (Sörensen et al., 2008), and with poorer problem-solving (Wetherell et al., 2002). Severe depression also impairs some aspects of memory and short-term planning among older adults (Blazer, 2009). Although depression is common with many chronic illnesses, the effect of depression on the likelihood of advance care planning has, to our knowledge, not been studied; however, patients with more anxiety and depressive symptoms *desire* more future discussions (Fakhri et al., 2016).

Understanding the potential effects of depression and personality on ARP is useful because interventions may need to be tailored to different personality types or styles of decision-making to have the desired effect. Policies that take into account the multi-level factors affecting individuals and the ways in which individual differences might affect adherence to recommendations are more likely to be effective.

Demographic, Socioeconomic Factors, and Family Factors in Aging-Related Preparation

Demographic factors are significant predictors of ARP in several domains, but their influence on ARP is often mediated through specific indicators of socioeconomic status (i.e., education, household income, access to social capital). In addition, some demographic factors are related to individuals' tolerance for risk, ability to tolerate ambiguity, retirement goal clarity, general planning practices (Ferraro, 1990; Jacobs-Lawson & Hershey, 2005; Stawski et al., 2005). Here we consider gender, socio-economic status, and family support.

Because women have a higher life expectancy than men (National Center for Health Statistics, 2020) and are often single in retirement (Tamborini et al., 2009), one would expect greater concern with financial planning. However, research into gender differences in retirement planning has had largely inconclusive results. Some studies show no differences (Hershey

& Mowen, 2000; Rosenkoetter & Garris, 2001; Reitzes & Mutran, 2004), but others do find small discrepancies, with women planning less (Jacobs-Lawson et al., 2004; Quick & Moen, 1998; Kim & Moen, 2001a; Kim & Moen, 2001b; Noone et al., 2010). Although women do more retirement planning compared to two decades ago, their overrepresentation in lower paid and nonunionized occupations with limited planning resources (O'Rand & Henretta, 1982; Kilty & Behling, 1986; Hayes & Parker, 1993; Muller et al., 2020), differences in financial literacy (Lusardi & Mitchell, 2008), lack of education about retirement (Perkins, 1995), and greater risk aversion (Agnew et al., 2003; Watson & McNaughton, 2007) may still contribute to some discrepancies. Women's financial retirement preparation is also related to home ownership, having longer planning horizons, and working for a large employer (Tamborini & Purcell, 2016).

Regarding PFC, women are more likely to have engaged in decision making (Mak & Sörensen, 2012; Sörensen & Pinquart, 2000c) and concrete preparation for long-term care (Black et al., 2008); their plans are more likely to involve specific long-term care services, like home care, housing arrangements, assisted living, and assistance with maintenance and lawn care (Robison et al., 2014). Although findings are not consistent regarding whether women do more ACP than men (Carr & Khodyakov, 2007; Carr et al., 2012), men are less likely to discuss their care preferences with others (Carr & Khodyakov, 2007).

Socio-economic status has been identified as important in most studies of ARP. Higher SES is related to greater retirement preparation (Noone et al., 2012), consideration of more housing choices (Robison et al., 2014), and PFC (Sörensen & Pinquart, 2000a, 2000c). This is likely due both to greater financial resources with which to plan, as well as more education on the available resources and ways to go about making plans. Consistent with this, advance care plans are most likely completed by older adults with higher education (Black et al., 2008; Triplett et al., 2008; Gerst & Burr, 2008) and income (Carr, 2012).

Family resources, such as more available family members, family financial assets, and social-emotional support allow older adults to plan more concretely (Sörensen & Pinquart, 2000a; Sörensen & Pinquart, 2000c; Song et al., 2016). Not having someone who can provide tangible assistance and living alone are both associated with less future care preparation (Black et al., 2008). But reliance on family may also suppress active preparation: avoidant planners are more likely to rely on adult children for assistance (Song et al., 2017). Experience caring for others enhances anticipation of future care needs, but not making specific plans (Finkelstein et al., 2012).

Even for elders with dementia, family caregivers are not well-prepared for end-of-life decision making (Gessert et al., 2001; Hirschman et al., 2008); yet when cognitive impairment renders elders unable to make decisions, fami-ly caregivers are generally called upon to make decisions about their care and treatment. Having supportive family relationships (Boerner et al., 2013) and even having grandchildren increases ACP (Gerst & Burr, 2008) and concern for family members may be a key motivation for older people to engage in ACP (Levi et al., 2010).

Community Factors in Aging-Related Preparation

At the community level, the extent to which aging services, transportation, housing options, and knowledge about those options are readily available influences older adults' ability to engage in ARP. These are often variable between rural, urban, and suburban living spaces. Also, community and cultural norms regarding the importance and acceptability of preparing for aging, and regional health systems' outreach for advance directives vary, and, thus, may influence adults' propensity to think about and engage in aging-related preparation. For example, norms regarding whether one should engage in PFC coming from family, culture, or the government can create social pressure to prepare for or <u>not</u> to mention future care. Family expectations for family caregiving can be unspoken or explicit and affect how elders engage in PFC. Family expectations may be unique to certain family systems (Spitze & Ward, 2000) or based in cultural views of eldercare (Delgadillo et al., 2004). Burton and Stack (1993) describe the concept of "kinscripts" that define how the caregiving role is perceived, who is responsible for family caregiving, and preferences for informal versus formal support (Stack & Burton, 1993), in African-American families, but potentially also in Asian-American (Pinquart & Sörensen, 2005), and Latino families (Delgadillo et al., 2004). Whether older adults plan for future care depends in part on such community-level factors, explaining, for example, higher rates of PFC among African Americans (Sörensen et al., 2014; Pinquart et al., 2003); this may be related to perceptions of greater caregiver availability in Black extended families (Roth et al., 2007) as well as higher community-level disease burden (Diez-Roux et al., 1997; Gary et al., 2008), which sensitizes African Americans to potential future care needs.

Elder care expectations based in culture and history may translate into filial obligation beliefs which are measurable at the individual level. These contribute to families' expectations of individual members to provide elder care (Ajrouch, 2005; Schans, 2008; Groger & Mayberry, 2001; Miyawaki, 2017; Guo et al., 2019; Wangmo, 2010). High filial obligation does not, however, necessarily translate into appropriate preparation or provision of care for the older adult. This may be a partial explanation for the finding that high filial norms are related to lower life satisfaction among some elders (Lowenstein et al., 2007). Filial obligation has been studied extensively, but how subjective norms contribute to engagement in ARP and planning for family or non-family care has not been assessed.

Local communities and their housing policies are critical in older adults' ability to plan for housing changes or for aging in place. Whereas choices of assisted living, housing modifications, and upscale nursing care are abundant for the wealthy, there is a lack of affordable, aging-suitable housing in many countries (Preston et al., 2019). Other community-level contributions to relocation plans include challenges of in-home management of increasing disability, access to, quality of, and range of aging services, insufficient public transportation, and distance from shopping and other daily needs (Hillcoat-Nallétamby & Ogg, 2014), concerns about neighborhood security, and lack of engagement with neighbors (Kearns & Parkes, 2003). Also, sense of community matters both to those older adults who decide to age in place (Jolanki & Villkoas, 2015) and those who move for the opportunity to reduce the burden of home maintenance and engage in meaningful activities in old age (Oswald & Wahl, 2005).

Community influences on ARP are also reflected in comparisons of ethnic minority communities to non-Hispanic Whites with regard to end-of-life planning. Whereas no differences in informal discussions about ACP are found, formal ACP is less common among racial/ethnic minority groups (Gerst & Burr, 2008; Choi et al., 2020). The relevance of race and ethnicity depends on other socio-economic, personal, and cultural variables, however. These include health status, being in treatment in hospital, or having more chronic illnesses as predictors of greater likelihood of ACP (Choi et al., 2020). Having greater education and health literacy, being older, and having more income are predictors of higher ACP among Latinx and Asian American groups (Hong et al., 2018). Homeownership increases the ACP engagement among Blacks. Cultural values and differences in priorities, spiritual beliefs, and lack of awareness or lack of knowledge about ACP may contribute to misunderstandings about ACP (Choi et al., 2020; Hong et al., 2018). In addition, Blacks often have had negative experiences the health care system resulting in mistrust and deterring their ACP engagement (Rhodes et al., 2017). In past studies, Latinx individuals were the least likely to participate in ACP (Eleazer et al., 1996), but recent works suggests they are open to end-of life discussions when offered the opportunity to discuss them in their preferred language with individualized, culturally competent materials (Maldonado et al., 2019). One key difference in the way communities of color and non-Hispanic whites approach aging-related preparation is that these communities are more likely to engage in family-centered collective processes in which opinions from family members about moving, care plans, and end of life are valued as much or even more than the elder's own preferences, and interdependence is valued more than autonomy and independence (Bullock, 2011).

Societal and Structural Factors in Aging-Related Preparation

Conceptions of ARP may look quite different across different countries with different social policies and cultures. Comparing older adults from Eastern and Western Germany and from Georgia and Utah, Pinquart et al. (2003) report that American respondents have the highest PFC scores. Although Germans and Americans are equally likely to avoid future care thoughts and worry that care needs might not be met, American elders are more likely to expect care, express awareness about those needs, gather information, decide on preferences, and make concrete plans. They also are more likely to report knowing their options and consider their home environment aging-appropriate. Furthermore, comparing within Eastern and Western Germany, East German elders were more likely to avoid planning for care, even seven years after reunification. Being less informed of possible options, they made fewer decisions, listed less-concrete plans, and were less satisfied with their planning. Many of these differences may be attributed to variations in policy and historical change. East Germans were embedded in a system of guaranteed (but mostly poor quality) nursing home care. With reunification, this system disappeared, and a population of elders already deprived of many life choices struggled to cope with rising nursing home costs and insecurities of social change. Compared the more individualistic policies in the U.S., Germany's social welfare state currently makes it possible to rely on public long-term care insurance which (partially) covers both nursing home and in-home care. These differences in national ethos on caring for the aging population, as well as differences in national dementia strategies that encourage assistance seeking and early diagnosis may also help families develop aging-related plans (Fortinsky & Downs, 2014).

Comparing adults in the U.S., Germany, and China, Kornadt et al. (2019) report that Germans and Americans claim more preparation than Chinese participants in all nine domains. This is likely due to family kinscripts and filial obligation beliefs within Chinese culture that proscribe care by family, but also differences between individualistic and communitarian societies. Chinese individuals who avoid future care preparation are more likely to rely on adult children for care (Song et al., 2016) and greater familism is related to family-focused care plans (Song et al., 2017). In contrast, awareness of future care needs and gathering information are related to an orientation toward service-focused (formal) care arrangements (Song et al., 2016). Consistent with Pinquart et al. (2003), Kornadt et al. (2019) find that with regard to health preparation, older American participants plan more than Germans elders, but not with regard to "emergency situations," which include health emergencies and end of life care.

Policies in the United States rely heavily on family care, self-financed formal care, or care covered by long-term care insurance, but that insurance has limited accessibility for individuals with limited financial means. Although long-term care is reliably covered by Medicaid for elders with limited income, considerable stress is placed on individuals in the middle-income bracket. As a result, for fear of bank-rupting their families, middle-class elders are often advised to transfer any wealth to children or trusts; "spending down" their wealth allows them to be eligible for Medicaid. This practice escalates Medicaid expenditures which were designed only for indigent elders and reduces seniors' choices among facilities that may not accept Medicaid. Elastic Medicaid eligibility rules, according to a report on California's Medi-Cal program, "desensitize the public to long-term care risks and costs, resulting in a false sense of security and entitlement" (Moses, 2011).

Unfortunately, programs and policies that increase pressure for planning for retirement and preparation for future care (Preston et al., 2019) are primarily focused on the cost of living and care, but not the clarification and selection of personal values preferences. Although maintaining one's current quality of life in spite of physical health declines is a primary activating and motivating factor for ARP, there is little incentive for middle-aged and older adults to struggle with issues that they find threatening. Even the acquisition of long-term care insurance may not have much relevance to middle-aged and older adults, if it does not assist them in maintaining quality of life as they define it—including resolving some of the paradoxes of care situations, such as maintaining privacy versus having regular access to one's social contacts or accessing intellectual and social stimulation versus remaining in familiar surroundings. Planning for financial coverage does not provide assurance that one's values will guide care decisions. Thus, "guaranteed care without a focus on care values may not suffice to maintain quality of life for older adults. Not much social encouragement exists, however, for older adults to clarify the type of care they prefer and why" (Sörensen, et al., 2011, p. 8).

Barriers to Aging-Related Preparation

Based on the findings reviewed above, a primary reason why individuals fail to prepare for age-related transitions is that they lack the financial and educational resources. In addition, knowledge of options plays a substantial role. Only a small minority of older adults can describe the financial coverage of long-term care, and those with lower incomes, who are married, and who have no living children are particularly vulnerable to long-term care financial literacy (Matzek & Stum, 2010). In the United States, the poorly developed private market for long-term care insurance, excludes many types of long-term care expenditures and is inaccessible to those who cannot afford high premiums (Brown & Finkelstein, 2004). Older adults often experience contradictions between wanting to plan and feeling unable to plan because available options are too costly.

A major barrier to ARP is the current structure of Medicare and Medicaid policy and its focus on acute medical care, rather than holistic principles of well-being. With regard to housing, we have suggested that by not planning for home modification or for moving to accommodate frailty (Adams & Rau, 2011; Tulle-Winton, 1999[2];

Gilroy, 2018), older adults may thwart their goals for "aging well." However, structural barriers to making plans for future housing are immense. In particular, the lack of age-friendly housing that does not segregate older adults against their will is lacking in most industrialized nations. Due to existing Medicaid policy, many lower income older individuals who are frail without being destitute may be unable to take advantage of more supportive housing opportunities, such as assisted living facilities (ALFs), because they cannot utilize Medicaid benefits as a form of payment at such facilities. This places such opportunities beyond the financial means of many middle-class elders. In addition, access to additional insurance may be limited due to lack of availability, even for those who can afford it. Aging in place may also not be a viable option, as communities may lack quality services due to insufficient oversight of direct care workers. Thus, even good planners may find they lack the services they need.[3] Other barriers to ARP have been explored in qualitative studies and relate to the stressful nature of preparation for future care. Protecting short-term well-being sometimes outweighs the perceived benefits of preparation (Craciun, & Flick, 2015; Sörensen & Pinquart 2000a; Pinquart & Sörensen, 2002a). Another barrier is the perception that contextual factors, such as national long-term care policies may change with little notice and thus render specific plans irrelevant in the future (Pinquart & Sörensen, 2002a), especially in times of social or economic instability.

Does Aging-Related Preparation Predict Better Outcomes?

The findings regarding benefits of ARP are somewhat inconsistent across the different domains of preparation.

Outcomes of Retirement Preparation

Although multiple studies support the beneficial effects of timely retirement preparation on physical and psychological health (Yeung, 2013; Yeung & Zhou, 2017), positive attitudes and adjustment to retirement (Reitzes & Mutran, 2004; Muratore & Earl, 2015), and higher life satisfaction (Topa et al., 2009; Noone et al., 2013), a systematic review by Barbosa et al. (2016) reports that retirement preparation by individuals is not among the strongest determinants of retirement adjustment. Retirement preparation is beneficial in only about half the studies reviewed; no difference is found in roughly 1/3 of studies, and negative effects of pre-retirement planning are observed in 8.7 % of the studies. Donaldson and colleagues (2010) suggest that physical and psychological health, the conditions under which a person exits the workforce, as well as their financial resources are more powerful predictors of adjustment, but that a higher personal sense of mastery mediates post- retirement planning. Although the inconsistencies between studies may be due in part to measures of planning behavior that focus on financial planning (Petkoska & Earl, 2009), there is some lack of clarity as to which kinds of preparation are beneficial under what circumstances (Donaldson et al., 2010). It is likely, though that retirement planning is not "complete" before the transition and that any early plans require modification over time.

Outcomes of Preparation for Future Care

Greater future care preparation can boost feelings of security and control (Pinquart & Sörensen, 2002a) which in turn contribute to life satisfaction (Kahana, et al., 2012). Care preparation, however, does not follow unitary patterns. Different styles of PFC are related to different short and long-term well-being outcomes. Styles of future care preparation have been identified in both qualitative and quantitative studies. (1) The "Avoiders" (Girling & Morgan, 2014; Sörensen, & Pinquart, 2000a, Steele et al., 2003) make up 5%-20% of the samples; they have particularly low scores in Awareness of Care Needs and Concrete Planning (Steele et al., 2003) and actively endorse not thinking about the future. Denton et al. (2004) also describe a group of "non-planners," who have experienced dramatic disruption in their lives and thus have abandoned making plans. Concurrent assessments of well-being suggest that avoiders have lower levels of concomitant depression outcomes (Steele et al., 2003), but a longitudinal study of older primary care patients shows that avoidance of future care planning is related to higher depression scores at 2-year follow-up (Sörensen et al., 2012). (2) The "Autonomous Care Planners" (34%,

Girling & Morgan, 2014) "Planners" (13.2%, Steele et al., 2003), and "Long-term planners" (45%, Sörensen & Pinquart, 2000a) display more worry, but also higher planning satisfaction than avoiders (Steele et al, 2003). Longitudinal data show that making concrete plans is associated with better outcomes: a lower likelihood of a depression diagnosis and lower anxiety scores after two years (Sörensen et al., 2012). (3) Individuals who engage in "Thinking without planning" (16%, Sörensen & Pinquart, 2000a) are aware of their preferences (20%, Girling & Morgan, 2014), but may agonize over their future (8.8%, Steele et al., 2003). No longitudinal data are available for the effects this planning style, but cross-sectionally it appears to be the most stressful (Steele, et al., 2003). (4) "Externally reliant care planners" (35%, Girling & Morgan, 2014) do not take an active role in planning details, and count on other individuals or agencies (e.g., the V.A., a religious order) to meet their needs. A parallel group with a much lower frequency, perhaps because of more stringent group criteria are "Consenters" (1.9%, Steele et al., 2003), who agree to other individuals' plans (cf. Maloney et al., 1996) and exhibit low levels of awareness but high levels of concrete planning; a comparable group of "Short-term planners" (24%, Sörensen & Pinquart, 2000a) focus on limited and more immediate needs, very general plans, or on saving money for unspecified future needs. In Steele et al.'s study, consenters are the most content with their plans and have low levels of worry. However, in Sörensen

and Pinquart's study (2000a) the short-term planners report that disruptions in their lives have led them to think of long-term planning as useless because of life's unpredictability. Taxonomies, such as the one above may be useful when considering policies directed at certain groups with different preparation styles and needs.

Outcomes of Advance Care Planning

The primary purpose for ACP is to ensure an elder's end-of-life wishes are known and respected, and to protect the elders' and their families' quality of life. Detering and colleagues (2010) report that individuals with assistance completing ACP have end of life wishes that are much more likely to be known and followed; their family members have significantly less stress, anxiety, and depression than control patients and their families. Their intervention positively affects both patient and family satisfaction (Detering et al., 2010). In a systematic review of 113 intervention articles, Brinkman-Stoppelenburg et al. (2014) find that ACP is associated with increased compliance with patients' end-of-life wishes, including avoidance of life-sustaining treatment (when not desired), a surge in use of hospice and palliative care among hospital patients, and less emergency hospitalization among nursing home patients.

In sum, longitudinal studies suggest the usefulness of pre-retirement planning for retirement adjustment, of certain types of preparation for future care for emotional well-being, and of ACP for a good death; the longitudinal effects of other domains of ARP have been studied less extensively. Preparing for changes and planning ahead may ameliorate adverse outcomes in old age, including limited future time perspective; for example, for leisure (Riddick & Stewart, 1994; Yeung, 2013), preventive health behaviors (Gessert et al., 2001; Kahana et al., 2012) and social planning (Yeung, 2013). Nevertheless, except for advance care planning among the very old, actual preparation behaviors are relatively low. It is clear that the positive effect of ARP is often enhanced by higher income and education, and greater problem-solving skill, but also linked to an increase in knowledge of options, services, and public resources. Particularly housing transitions (or aging in place) can be improved dramatically with access to resources; the effect of housing decisions and transitions on psychological well-being is still under-researched.

Interventions to Enhance ARP and Policy Implications

The World Health Organization (WHO, 2015) has recommended five areas that need to be addressed by policy, including (1) devoting effort to healthy aging that requires developing a cohesive set of targeted policies that benefit older adults; (2) developing health system policies that align with the needs of older adults; (3) establishing mechanisms to provide chronic disease care for older adults; (4) creating environments that adapt to older adults' needs; and (5) improving, measuring, understanding, and

encouraging the study of factors that contribute to the care and well-being of older adults. As noted above, individual differences in ARP can be attributed to psychological factors, family and community factors, policies, and cultural orientations regarding the necessity and usefulness of planning and the obligations of family, but policies both determine individual actions and affect government expenditures.

State and national long-term care policies differ in the extent to which they support and/or expect families to prepare for retirement, prepare for and provide all care, partial care, or no care, develop advance directives, not to mention engage in leisure or social preparation. In addition, there is a need for informal caregivers to partner with health care providers and acquire adequate skills to adapt to their role as the disease trajectory of care recipients' changes over time. The expectation among healthcare providers and payers is that informal caregivers (family and friends) will provide caregiving services in the home. Unfortunately, there is rarely a meaningful discussion on whether informal caregivers are available, willing, or able to take up the responsibility, for example after hospital discharge (Schulz et al., 2018); about half of all family caregivers report having no choice in taking on the caregiving role. Only about a third of the family caregivers indicate that they have been contacted by the health care providers to inquire what support they need in order to provide care; 84% of family caregivers indicate that they need more caregiving training (Lee et al., 2020).

Since the evidence suggests that older adults tend to engage in inadequate ARP for their own care, and family members often take on care without proper preparation, new policies may be required that better integrate other family members, such as adult children, into the preparation process.

In this context, federal and state governments must recognize the needs of family caregivers who deliver care (Lee et al., 2020). These efforts are obstructed by unresolved problems of how family members, the private sector, and government would pay for caregiving expenses (Gaugler & Kane, 2015). At the federal level, the 2018 Recognize, Assist, Include, Support and Engage (RAISE; Cacchione, 2019) act was passed into law in order to implement a national strategy to support family caregiving. Additionally, new policies of the Centers for Medicare and Medicaid Services and others were also implemented to support family caregivers for people living with serious illnesses (Friedman & Rizzolo, 2016). Despite these initiatives, caregivers' services are currently not adequately supported by policy and practice (Schulz et al., 2020).

We do not, however, think it is reasonable to assume that family members will assume responsibilities for older adults through the sheer force of moral exhortation. Rather, incentivizing assistance with ARP may be required. This could involve providing a guide for adult children through state-level campaigns to initiate discussions about aging-related preparation with their parents, similar to the campaigns for

Advance Care Planning and Medical Orders for Life-Sustaining Treatment (Compassion and Support, 2020) that have successfully increased completion of ACP forms (e.g., in New York State; Bomba & Orem 2015; Bomba et al., 2011). However, when considering family-centered approaches to caregiving, researchers and policymakers should be mindful of the manner in which such approaches may differentially impact male and female family members, leading to further challenges related to social justice and equity (DePasquale et al., 2015; Schmid et al., 2011).

Furthermore, family members are not the only social actors who are well positioned to assist with aging-related preparation. Employers, too, can contribute to ARP either by supporting aging employees directly or engaging family members who support them. Aging-related preparation has not been publicly emphasized and, thus, few know how to go about it. This lack of awareness should be rectified through a consistent and extended public health campaign (because campaign success is increased by the application of multiple repetitions (Wakefield et al., 2010)). The campaign should not only educate the public about the need for ARP, but focus on clarification of interests and values, rather than purely on financial or medical aspects of long-term care. Concurrently, key resources that explain options and services must be available, such as the AARPs resource guide "Planning for Long-term Care" or Minnesota's "Care to Plan" website for dementia caregivers (Gaugler et al. 2016), but in multiple languages and with greater attention to accessibility for the visually impaired and those with limited literacy, and with a broader scope than caregiving or long-term care.

Governmental shifts to encouraging individual pre-retirement financial planning are frequently tied to attempts to reduce social programs without addressing the structural barriers to preparation for late life (Preston et al., 2019). Thus, a societal focus on "shaping your own future" is a double-edged sword; on the one hand it could encourage greater ARP across all domains of lifestyle planning, potentially increasing older adults' control over their life circumstances and quality of life. On the other hand, it could marginalize groups who lack the necessary resources, skill, or predisposition to plan. The evidence reviewed here, therefore, suggests that individual pre-retirement financial planning is not a suitably effective replacement for social programs and that adequate ARP must be a joint and integrated effort involving all stakeholders, such as the state, the individual, the family, and the community. In the next section we discuss interventions to increase ARP, focusing only on pre-retirement, Preparation for Future Care, and Housing Preparation, as the field of ACP is already replete with effective interventions (Bryant, et al., 2019).

Interventions for Improved Retirement Planning

Pre-retirement planning programs, which originated during the 1950s at several large Midwestern universities, are voluntary (Hayes & Parker, 1993) and usually limited to the financial aspects and immediate post-employment period. Few are more comprehensive in scope, addressing health, leisure, finances, social relations. They are offered as group programs or individual counseling by large employers and—on-line and in written format—by the Social Security Administration and the Department of Labor. Often these programs are oriented to a male career model, and often poorly attended by women (Hayes & Parker, 1993). Based on the inconsistent findings regarding the effectiveness of preretirement programs in improving retirement adjustment (Barbosa et al., 2016), it is likely that preretirement programs require an overhaul (see Box 3). Consistent with our recommendations in the previous section, these programs would benefit not only from a greater focus on enhancing mastery and providing coaching for how to negotiate healthy retirement conditions (Donaldson et al., 2010), but also from addressing the entire range of ARP domains.

BOX 3: Policy Recommendations for Improved Retirement Planning:

- A guaranteed retirement income that will cover basic needs. Retirees should not have to trade purchasing food for getting their medication. At that level of survival, planning becomes a luxury (Denton et al., 2004).

- The implementation of pay equity is crucial for women's ARP.

- Additional opportunities for education and training for women in midlife could contribute to for women's independence in later life.

- The need to plan for a longer period of retirement should be anticipated, given greater longevity.

- Policies need to address the increasingly precarious nature of a workforce subject to short term contracts, part-time and casual employment, that add to more difficulty to the task of saving for retirement, particularly for older women.

- Greater flexibility for older workers approaching retirement to improve the exit conditions, including job sharing, job transfers, sabbaticals, and eliminating forced early retirement, thus increasing employee levels of control in the retirement decision (Quine et al., 2007).

- Because employees may be reluctant to initiate discussions about retirement, culturally sanctioned options for such discussions should be provided by employers. Planning for aging might be integrated into vocational/professional continuing education. Middle-aged workers could receive information about assisting aging parents and begin the preparation process for their own later years.

- HR departments should focus on supporting mastery and employees' self-efficacy beliefs about their ability to plan for positive outcomes using control enhancing experiences and modeling, thus building resilience.

Interventions for Preparation for Future Care

Several programmatic attempts have been made to enhance individual long-term care preparation. A free program offered through State Departments of Aging to encourage long-term care preparation, such as a long-term care consultation service had poor attendance (McGrew, 2006). A six-state campaign to induce individuals to consider long-term care insurance involving a letter from the State's governor inviting adults over 55 to order a long-term care planning kit generated a response rate of less than 8% (Long Term Care Group, Inc. & LifePlans, Inc. for U.S. Department of Health and Human Services, 2006; Tell & Cutler, 2011). The lack of response to these efforts can be attributed to several factors. First, offering such programs to the 55+ population at large may lack the context older adults need to recognize the need to plan. As mentioned above, functional status losses, need for care, and residential transitions are stressful topics often avoided. In acute health crises there may be an immediate need for action (and therefore ordering a planning kit is unhelpful); if needs are not acute, arousal of negative emotions (Aspinwall & Taylor, 1997) may prevent proactive engagement and foster avoidance, since the discussions are seen as "not yet relevant." Second, one size fits all programs are unlikely to resonate with individuals from different life stages, cultural groups, resource rich or resource poor community environments. Consistent with our recommendations above, programs offered through the community should strive to incorporate the entire family and especially adult children, if available, into the preparation process. A concrete example of how employers can support employees with aging family members is by offering them paid time off in addition to vacation and sick leave. Admittedly, given current norms and economic circumstances this possibility is unlikely to be realized without a significant shift in attitudes, which suggests that in addition to recommending specific policies, advocates should also work towards shifting the Overton window (the range of policies deemed acceptable by the general public) with respect to paid leave (Mackinac Center for Public Policy, 2019).

Third, many older adults, having retired years ago, are not prepared for the new types of problems they are facing, and may lack the information, skills, health literacy, and persistence to accomplish preparation for potential care needs. Thus, programs offered through the community must be tailored to the needs of the individuals within them, taking into account the local resources. One such program, recently introduced by Lee et al. (2019) focuses on encouraging future planning in six areas: housing, medical care, nutrition needs, health incidents, financial needs, and care needs in a 2-session group program administered by cooperative extension program facilitators. An increase in planning activities in pre-post tests suggests that the format is promising. However, a drawback of programs that explicitly invite individuals to learn about future planning is that the attendees are self-selected and that those who need the programs the most often do not attend.

Another intervention to enhance preparation for age-related changes, specifically for older adults with progressive vision loss, has focused on assisting older adults in preparing for future care using a "stealth" approach to future planning. Based on a clinical trial of the program with Macular Degeneration Patients (Sörensen et al., 2015) the project, Resilience-Building Intervention to prevent Late-life Depression with Vision Loss (REBUILD-VL), harnesses the concerns and needs of older adults with vision loss to then interject content and training about future care preparation. After four group classes about different aspects of vision loss, participants engage in "resilience building coaching" (based on problem solving therapy approaches; Areán et al., 2020; Mynors-Wallis et al., 1995), focusing initially on current issues, such as transportation, personal relationships, lack of social connection. After acquiring this systematic way to approach and (at least partially) solve problems, they proceed to discussing potential *future* issues, such as anticipated housing transitions, replacing valued activities after losing vision, or needing in-home assistance. Pilot work suggests an improvement in problem-solving skill (Point-du Jour & Sörensen, 2009) as well as increases in Decision Making and Concrete Planning (Sörensen et al., 2008; 2014; Sörensen, 2019), compared to a comparison group that conducted a life review. This dual strategy of building problem solving skills and trust, before focusing on topics that are more anxiety-laden could translate to other populations.

Interventions for Housing Preparation

Preparation for housing transitions or aging in place has been very limited in the public forum, compared to income and health (Pynoos, 2018). Because there is a shortage of affordable, accessible, and supportive housing for older adults, many elders are unable to identify the "ideal" living situation that would help them maintain independence, health and everyday competence. Although not an intervention to enhance preparation for housing transitions, a program by Szanton and colleagues (2011), The Community Aging in Place, Advancing Better Living for Elders (CAPABLE) deserves mention. This program allows older individuals with low income and with difficulties

performing activities of daily living coordinated access to occupational therapy (up to 6 visits), nurses (up to 4 visits), and handyman repairs (up to $1,300). Compared to attention-control visits, the intervention group shows reduced difficulty with Activities of Daily Living (ADLs) and instrumental ADLs, better self-reported quality of life, and lower risk of falls. Thus, making health care and home maintenance resources more accessible increases the older adults' ability to age in place. Although not explicitly geared toward engaging the older adults in ARP activities, the program assists participants to identify and prioritize goals (such as pain and depression management), construct behavioral plans, modify and repair their built environment to decrease fall risk, increase mobility, and ultimately prevent nursing home placement, while supporting them in their wish to age in place in the residential environment that they know and value.

Conclusion

As increasing numbers of the Baby Boomer cohort retire, interventions and policies need to be built around an understanding of the factors that promote effective Aging-Related Preparation. Current policies make finding age-friendly housing, long-term care, and adequate retirement income a personal responsibility that requires middle-aged and older adults to plan, save, invest, and insure themselves (Moses, 2011; Preston et al., 2019). In our view the effectiveness of the personal responsibility model of preparation has not been vindicated by the literature. Society's interest in taking care of its aging population would be better served by adopting the language of rights to include older adults' basic needs in order to refocus aging-related preparation as a way to flourish (Gilroy, 2008) rather than merely survive. This would further serve the aims of social justice by partially rectifying systemic inequalities, which otherwise are amplified in late life. As mentioned above, the most disenfranchised societal groups often have the least internal and external resources with which to prepare for aging; thus, they are least likely to attain their goals for old age. Applying more cultural and social pressure for family-based care preparation without providing scaffolding and resources is likely to fail both the individuals affected and the goal of government savings. For this reason, we reiterate the need for an integrated approach that involves the state, the family, and the community.

Framed in such social justice and community-based terms, we see that the majority of interventions may be predicated on a set of unexamined cultural assumptions that are nevertheless accepted as fact in individualistic cultures. Whereas mastery, planning and problem-solving skills, personality, knowledge and beliefs play a role in ARP, the larger socio-cultural context creates the structure within which personal goals can be realized or are perceived as unrealistic. *Knowledge* of resources is not sufficient without *access* to adequate financial, housing, transportation, and medical resources, which provide a basis for effective preparation. Because the majority of interventions

to enhance ARP are based on working with individuals on their personal goals, plans, knowledge of resources, and coping skills, we as interventionists are maintaining the status quo regarding the relationship of the aging individual to society. Thus, despite the often intuitive appeal of the individual-based approach to interventionists working in individualistic cultures, the literature suggests that a more communitarian ethos that shifts ARP responsibility from the individual to the societal level could overcome more barriers to preparing for age-related changes. Consequently, interventionists might critically assess and advocate for a new relationship of the aging individual to society. A practical example, based on Szanton et al.'s (2011) work would be to make public funds available for home modifications, allowing older adults to prepare for aging in place with more confidence. Other examples of systemic/policy changes that would enhance effective ARP are shown in Box 2.

While adults in late middle-age and the "third age" are concerned with preparing for financial and role changes associated with retirement, older adults may be tasked with managing increasing chronic conditions that affect mobility and function, while also trying to afford quality housing, and continuing to pursue their personal goals in the areas of family and social relationships, leisure, work and volunteering. National and state policies, as well as future-oriented age-friendly communities can create the environmental, economic, and social contexts that allow older people to identify, plan for, and pursue their goals. New solutions at the systems level are needed to assist adults with integrating preparation and planning for age-related changes. Planners need to be able to access information about health conditions, care options, financial supports, and available aging services to convert aging-related goals into concrete plans, if ARP is to be realistic.

References

AARP Public Policy Institute & National Alliance for Caregiving (2015, June). Caregiving in the U.S.: Research Report. Retrieved from https://www.aarp.org/content/dam/aarp/ppi/2015/caregiving-in-the-united-states-2015-report-revised.pdf

AARP (2010). Planning for Long-Term Care: Your Resource Guide. Retrieved from https://assets.aarp.org/www.aarp.org_/cs/health/ltc_resource_guide.pdf

Adams, G.A., & Rau, B.L. (2011). Putting off tomorrow to do what you want today: planning for retirement. *The American Psychologist, 66*,180–192. doi:10.1037/a0022131

Age Wave & Harris Interactive (2010) America Talks: Protecting Our Families' Financial Futures. Retrieved from https://www.genworth.com/dam/Americas/US/PDFs/Consumer/corporate/America_Talks.pdf

Agnew, J., Balduzzi, P., & Sunden, A. (2003). Portfolio choice and trading in a large 401 (k) plan. *American Economic Review, 93*(1), 193-215.

Ajrouch, K. J. (2005). Arab-American immigrant elders' views about social support. *Ageing & Society, 25*(5), 655-673.

Allen, R. S., Oliver, J. S., Eichorst, M. K., Mieskowski, L., Payne-Foster, P., & Sörensen, S. (2019). Preparation and planning for future care in the Deep South: Adapting a validated tool for cultural sensitivity. *The Gerontologist, 59*(6), e643-e652. doi:10.1093/geront/gny102

Ameriks, J., Caplin, A., & Leahy, J. (2002). Wealth accumulation and the propensity to plan. National Bureau of Economic Research, Working Paper #8920.

Ameriks, J., Caplin, A., & Leahy, J. (2003). Wealth accumulation and the propensity to plan. *The Quarterly Journal of Economics, 118*(3), 1007-1047.

Apouye, B. H. (2018). Preparation for old age in France: The roles of preferences and expectations. *The Journal of the Economics of Ageing, 12*, 15-23.

Areán, P. A., Raue, P., Mackin, R. S., Kanellopoulos, D., McCulloch, C., & Alexopoulos, G. S. (2010). Problem-solving therapy and supportive therapy in older adults with major depression and executive dysfunction. *American Journal of Psychiatry, 167*(11), 1391-1398.

Aspinwall, L.G. (1997). Where planning meets coping: proactive coping and the detection and management of potential stressors. In: S.L. Friedman & E.K. Scholnick (Eds.), *The developmental psychology of planning: Why, how, and when do we plan?* (pp. 285-320). London: Lawrence Erlbaum Associates, Publishers.

Aspinwall, L.G., & Taylor, S.E. (1997). A stitch in time: self-regulation and proactive coping. *Psychological Bulletin, 121,* 417-436.

Aspinwall, L. G. (2005). The psychology of future-oriented thinking: From achievement to proactive coping, adaptation, and aging. *Motivation and emotion, 29*(4), 203-235.

Baltes, P. B., & Baltes, M. M. (1990). Psychological perspectives on successful aging: The model of selective optimization with compensation. In P. B. Baltes & M. M. Baltes (Eds.), *Successful aging: Perspectives from the behavioral sciences* (pp. 1–34). Cambridge: Cambridge Univ. Press.

Baltes, B. B., Rudolph, C. W., & Bal, A. C. (2012). A review of aging theories and modern work perspectives. *The Oxford handbook of work and aging,* 117-136.

Baltes, P.B., & Smith, J. (2003). New frontiers in the future of aging: from successful aging of the young old to the dilemmas of the fourth age. *Gerontology, 49,*123–135. doi:10.1159/000067946

Baltes, P.B., Smith, J., & Staudinger, U.M. (1992). Wisdom and successful aging. In: Sonderegger TB (ed) *Nebraska symposium on motivation 1991: Psychology and Aging. Current theory and research in motivation.* University of Nebraska Press, Lincoln, pp 123–167

Barbosa, L. M., Monteiro, B., & Murta, S. G. (2016). Retirement adjustment predictors—A systematic review. *Work, Aging and Retirement, 2*(2), 262-280.

Barlow, M., Wrosch, C., Heckhausen, J., & Schulz, R. (2016). Control Strategies for Managing Physical Health Problems in Old Age. *Perceived control: Theory, research, and practice in the first 50 years,* 281.

Barrett, L. (2014). Home and Community Preferences of the 45+ Population 2014. Washington, DC: AARP Research Center.

Begley, J., & Lambie-Hanson, L. (2015). The home maintenance and improvement behaviors of older adults in Boston. *Housing Policy Debate, 25*(4), 754-781.

Berg, C. A., Strough, J., Calderone, K., Meegan, S. P., & Sansone, C. (1997). Planning to prevent everyday problems from occurring. *The developmental psychology of planning: Why, how, and when do we plan*, 209-236.

Bernheim, B. D., Skinner, J., & Weinberg, S. (1997). What accounts for the variation in retirement wealth among US households? (No. w6227). National Bureau of Economic Research.

Beshears, J, Choi, J.J., Laibson D., & Madrian, B. (2008). The importance of default options for retirement saving outcomes: Evidence from the United States. In S.J. Kay and T. Sinha (Eds)., *Lessons from Pensions Reform in the Americas (pp. 59-87.)* Oxford: Oxford University Press,

Black, K., Reynolds, S. L., & Osman, H. (2008). Factors associated with advance care planning among older adults in southwest Florida. *Journal of Applied Gerontology, 27*(1), 93-109.

Blackwood, D. H., Walker, D., Mythen, M. G., Taylor, R. M., & Vindrola-Padros, C. (2019). Barriers to advance care planning with patients as perceived by nurses and other healthcare professionals: A systematic review. *Journal of Clinical Nursing, 28*(23-24), 4276-4297.

Blekesaune, M., Skirbekk, V. (2012). Can personality predict retirement behaviour? A longitudinal analysis combining survey and register data from Norway. *The European Journal of Ageing, 9*(3),199-206. Published 2012 Jan 10. doi:10.1007/s10433-011-0212-6

Boerner, K., Carr, D., & Moorman, S. (2013). Family relationships and advance care planning: Do supportive and critical relations encourage or hinder planning? *Journals of Gerontology Series B, 68*(2), 246-256.

Bogetic, Z., Onder, H., Onal, A., Skrok, E. A., Schwarz, A., & Winkler, H. (2015). Fiscal policy issues in the aging societies. *Macroeconomics & Fiscal Management Discussion Paper Series*, (1). In P.A. Linley & S. Joseph (Eds.) *Positive psychology in practice*. Wiley, Hoboken, pp 165–178.

Bomba, P. A., & Orem, K. (2015). Lessons learned from New York's community approach to advance care planning and MOLST. *The Annals of Palliative Medicine, 4*(1), 10-21.

Bomba, P. A., Morrissey, M. B., & Leven, D. C. (2011). Key role of social work in effective communication and conflict resolution process: Medical Orders for Life-Sustaining Treatment (MOLST) program in New York and shared medical decision making at the end of life. *Journal of Social Work in End-of-Life & Palliative Care, 7*(1), 56-82

Brunstein, J. C., Schultheiss, O. C., & Maier, G. W. (1999). The pursuit of personal goals. *Action & self-development*, 169-196.

Brandtstädter. J., & Rothermund, K. (2003). Intentionality and time in human development and aging: compensation and goal adjustment in changing developmental contexts. In: Staudinger UM, Lindenberger U (eds) *Understanding human development: Dialogues with lifespan psychology.* Kluwer Academic Publishers, Dordrecht, pp 105–124

Brandtstädter, J. (2009). Goal pursuit and goal adjustment: Self-regulation and intentional self-development in changing developmental contexts. *Advances in Life Course Research, 14*(1-2), 52-62.

Brandtstädter, J., & Rothermund, K. (2002). The life-course dynamics of goal pursuit and goal adjustment: A two-process framework. *Developmental review, 22*(1), 117-150.

Brandstätter, V., Lengfelder, A., & Gollwitzer, P. M. (2001). Implementation intentions and efficient action initiation. *Journal of personality and social psychology, 81*(5), 946.

Brinkman-Stoppelenburg, A., Rietjens, J. A., & Van der Heide, A. (2014). The effects of advance care planning on end-of-life care: a systematic review. *Palliative medicine, 28*(8), 1000-1025.

Bryant, J., Turon, H., Waller, A., Freund, M., Mansfield, E., & Sanson-Fisher, R. (2019). Effectiveness of interventions to increase participation in advance care planning for people with a diagnosis of dementia: a systematic review. *Palliative medicine, 33*(3), 262-273.

Bucher-Koenen, T., & Lusardi, A. (2011). *Financial literacy and retirement planning in Germany* (No. w17110). National Bureau of Economic Research.

Buck, G. B. (1926). Baltimore's new retirement system. *National Municipal Review, 15,* 454.

Bullock, K. (2011).The influence of culture on end-of-life decision making. *Journal of Social Work and End of Life Palliative Care, 7,*83–98.943.

Burton, L. M., & Stack, C. B. (1993). Conscripting kin: Reflections on family, generation, and culture. *The politics of pregnancy: Adolescent sexuality and public policy.* (pp. 174-185). New Haven, CT: Yale University Press.

Byles, J., Curryer, C., Vo, K., Forder, P., Loxton, D., & McLaughlin, D. (2018). Changes in housing among older women: Latent class analysis of housing patterns in older Australian women. *Urban Studies, 55*(4), 917-934.

Cacchione, P. Z. (2019). The Recognize, Assist, Include, Support and Engage (RAISE) Family Caregivers Act. *Clinical Nursing Research, 28*(8), 907-910.

https://doi.org/10.1177/1054773819876130

Camhi, S. L., Mercado, A. F., Morrison, R. S., Du, Q., Platt, D. M., August, G. I., & Nelson, J. E. (2009). Deciding in the dark: advance directives and continuation of treatment in chronic critical illness. *Critical care medicine, 37*(3), 919.

Cantor, N., Norem, J., Langston, C., Zirkel, S., Fleeson, W., & Cook-Flannagan, C. (1991). Life tasks and daily life experience. *Journal of personality, 59*(3), 425-451.

Carver, L. F., Beamish, R., Phillips, S. P., & Villeneuve, M. (2018). A scoping review: Social participation as a cornerstone of successful aging in place among rural older adults. *Geriatrics, 3*(4), 75.

Carr D. & Khodyakov, D. (2007). End-of-life health care planning among young-old adults: An assessment of psychosocial influences. *The Journals of Gerontology Series B: Psychological Sciences and Social Sciences, 62*, S135–S141.

Carr, D. (2012). The social stratification of older adults' preparations for end of life health care. *Journal of Health and Social Behavior, 53*, 297–312.

Carr, D., Moorman, S. M., & Boerner, K. (2013). End-of-life planning in a family context: Does relationship quality affect whether (and with whom) older adults plan? *Journals of Gerontology Series B, 68*(4), 586-592.

Carrese, J. A., Mullaney, J. L., Faden, R. R., & Finucane, T. E. (2002). Planning for death but not serious future illness: qualitative study of housebound elderly patients. *British Medical Journal, 325*(7356), 125-127.

Carstensen, G., Rosberg, B., Mc Kee, K. J., & Åberg, A. C. (2019). Before evening falls: Perspectives of a good old age and healthy ageing among oldest-old Swedish men. *Archives of gerontology and geriatrics, 82*, 35-44.

Carstensen, L.L. (2006). The influence of a sense of time on human development. *Science, 312*, 1913–1915. doi:10.1126/science.1127488

Carstensen, L. L., Fung, H. H., & Charles, S. T. (2003). Socioemotional selectivity theory and the regulation of emotion in the second half of life. *Motivation and emotion, 27*(2), 103-123.

Carstensen, L.L., Isaacowitz, D.M., & Charles, S.T. (1999). Taking time seriously. A theory of socioemotional selectivity. *American Psychologist, 54*, 165–181. doi:10.1037/0003-066X.54.3.165

Carver, L. F., Beamish, R., Phillips, S. P., & Villeneuve, M. (2018). A scoping review: Social participation as a cornerstone of successful aging in place among rural older adults. *Geriatrics, 3*(4), 75.

Chan, M. C., Chung, E. K., & Yeung, D. Y. (2020). Attitudes toward retirement drive the effects of retirement preparation on psychological and physical well-being of Hong Kong Chinese retirees over time. *The International Journal of Aging and Human Development*, 91415020926843. doi:10.1177/0091415020926843

Chen, Y., Lee, Y., Pethtel, O. L., Gutowitz, M. S., & Kirk, R. M. (2012). Age differences in goal concordance, time use, and well-being. *Educational Gerontology, 38*(11), 742-752. doi:10.1080/03601277.2011.645424

Choi, S., McDonough, I. M., Kim, M., & Kim, G. (2020). The association between the number of chronic health conditions and advance care planning varies by race/ethnicity. *Aging & Mental Health, 24*(3), 453-463.

Cohen-Mansfield, J., Droge, J. A., & Billig, N. (1992). Factors influencing hospital patients' preferences in the utilization of life-sustaining treatments. *The Gerontologist, 32*(1), 89-95.

Compassion and Support (2020). Excellus BlueCross Blue Shield. Retrieved from https://compassionandsupport.org/

Court, D. Farrell, D. & Forsyth, J.E. (2007). Serving aging baby boomers. *McKinsey Quarterly, 4*, 102-113.

Craciun, C., & Flick, U. (2015). "I want to be 100 years old, but I smoke too much": Exploring the gap between positive aging goals and reported preparatory actions in different social circumstances. *Journal of aging studies, 35*, 49-54.

Craik, F. I., & Bialystok, E. (2006). Planning and task management in older adults: Cooking breakfast. *Memory & Cognition, 34*(6), 1236-1249. Doi. org/10.3758/BF03193268

Cross, S., & Markus, H. (1991). Possible selves across the life span. *Human development, 34*(4), 230-255.

Degenholtz, H.B, Arnold, R.A, Meisel, A., & Lave, J.R. (2002). Persistence of racial disparities in advance care plan documents among nursing home residents. The *Journal of the American Geriatric Society, 50*, 378-381.

Delgadillo, L., Sörensen, S. & Coster. D.C. (2004). An exploratory study of factors related to preparation for future care among older Hispanics in Utah. *Journal of Family and Economic Issues, 25* (1): 51-78. https://link.springer.com/content/pdf/10.1023/B:JEEI.0000016723.31676.fe.pdf

Denton, M. A., Kemp, C. L., French, S., Gafni, A., Joshi, A., Rosenthal, C. J., Davies, S. (2004). Reflexive planning for later life. *Canadian Journal on Aging, 23*, S71–S82. doi:10.1353/cja.2005.0031

DePasquale, N., Polenick, C. A., Davis, K. D., Moen, P., Hammer, L. B., & Almeida, D. M. (2015;2017;). The psychosocial implications of managing work and family caregiving roles: Gender differences among information technology professionals. *Journal of Family Issues, 38*(11), 1495-1519. doi:10.11 77/0192513x15584680

Desai, M.M., Lentzner, H.R. Weeks, J.D. (2001). Unmet need for personal assistance with activities of daily living among older adults, *The Gerontologist, 41*(1), 82–88. https://doi.org/10.1093/geront/41.1.82

Detering, K. M., Buck, K., Ruseckaite, R., Kelly, H., Sellars, M., Sinclair, C., ... & Nolte, L. (2019). Prevalence and correlates of advance care directives among older Australians accessing health and residential aged care services: Multicentre audit study. *BMJ open, 9*(1).

Detering, K. M., Hancock, A. D., Reade, M. C., & Silvester, W. (2010). The impact of advance care planning on end of life care in elderly patients: Randomised controlled trial. *British Medical Journal*, 340, c1345. doi.org/10.1136/bmj. c1345

Dexter, P. R., Wolinsky, F. D., Gramelspacher, G. P., Zhou, X., Eckert, G. J., Waisburd, M., & Tierney, W. M. (1998). Effectiveness of computer-generated reminders for increasing discussions about advance directives and completion of advance directive forms: A randomized, controlled trial. Annals of Internal Medicine, 128(2), 102-110. doi:10.7326/0003-4819-128-2-199801150-00005

Diez-Roux, A. V., Nieto, F. J., Muntaner, C., Tyroler, H. A., Comstock, G. W., Shahar, E., ... & Szklo, M. (1997). Neighborhood environments and coronary heart disease: a multilevel analysis. *American journal of epidemiology, 146*(1), 48-63.

Dixon, J., Karagiannidou, M., & Knapp, M. (2018). The effectiveness of advance care planning in improving end-of-life outcomes for people with dementia and their carers: A systematic review and critical discussion. *Journal of Pain and Symptom Management, 55*(1), 132-150.

Ditto, P. H., Danks, J. H., Smucker, W. D., Bookwala, J., Coppola, K. M., Dresser, R., ... & Zyzanski, S. (2001). Advance directives as acts of communication: a randomized controlled trial. *Archives of Internal Medicine, 161*(3), 421-430.

Dohmen, T., Falk, A., Huffman, D., Sunde, U., Schupp, J., & Wagner, G. G. (2011). Individual risk attitudes: Measurement, determinants, and behavioral consequences. *Journal of the European Economic Association, 9*(3), 522-550.

Donaldson, T., Earl, J. K., & Muratore, A. M. (2010). Extending the integrated model of retirement adjustment: Incorporating mastery and retirement planning. *Journal of Vocational Behavior, 77*(2), 279-289.

Earl, J.K. & Archibald H. (2014) Retirement planning is more than just the accumulation of resources. *European Journal of Management, 14,* 21-36.

Ekerdt, D. J., Hackney, J., Kosloski, K., & DeViney, S. (2001). Eddies in the stream: The prevalence of uncertain plans for retirement. *The Journals of Gerontology. Series B, Psychological Sciences and Social Sciences, 56*(3), S162-S170. doi:10.1093/geronb/56.3.S162

Ejaz, F. K. (2000). Predictors of advance directives in institutionalized elderly. *Journal of Gerontological Social Work, 33*(4), 67-89.

Eleazer, G.P., Hornung, C.A., & Egbert, C.B., et al. (1996). The relationship between ethnicity and advance directives in a frail older population. *Journal American Geriatrics Society, 44,* 938.

Elliott, R. (2003). Executive functions and their disorders: Imaging in clinical neuroscience. *British medical bulletin, 65*(1), 49-59.

Emanuel, L. L., Emanuel, E. J., Barry, M. J., Stoeckle, J. D., & Ettelson, L. M. (1991). Advance directives for medical care—A case for greater use. *The New England Journal of Medicine, 324*(13), 889-895. doi:10.1056/NEJM199103283241305

Emmons, R. A. (1989). The personal striving approach to personality. *Goal Concepts in Personality and Social Psychology,* 87-126.

Emmons, R. A. (1999). *The psychology of ultimate concerns: Motivation and spirituality in personality.* Guilford Press.

Erickson, M. A., Krout, J., Ewen, H., & Robison, J. (2006). Should I stay or should I go? Moving plans of older adults. *Journal of Housing for the Elderly, 20*(3), 5-22.

Evans, L., Ekerdt, D. J., & Bosse, R. (1985). Proximity to retirement and anticipatory involvement: Findings from the normative aging study. *Journal of Gerontology, 40*(3), 368-374. https://doi.org/10.1093/geronj/40.3.368

Fakhri, S., Engelberg, R. A., Downey, L., Nielsen, E. L., Paul, S., Lahdya, A. Z., ... & Curtis, J. R. (2016). Factors affecting patients' preferences for and actual discussions about end-of-life care. *Journal of pain and symptom management, 52*(3), 386-394.

Femia, E. E., Zarit, S. H., & Johansson, B. (2001). The disablement process in very late life: a study of the oldest-old in Sweden. *The Journals of Gerontology Series B: Psychological Sciences and Social Sciences, 56*(1), P12-P23.

Ferraro, K. F. (1990). Cohort analysis of retirement preparation, 1974–1981. *Journal of Gerontology, 45*(1), S21-S31.

Finkelstein, E. S., Reid, M. C., Kleppinger, A., Pillemer, K., & Robison, J. (2012). Are baby boomers who care for their older parents planning for their own future long-term care needs? *Journal of Aging & Social Policy, 24*(1), 29-45.

Finlayson, M., & Van Denend, T. (2003). Experiencing the loss of mobility: perspectives of older adults with MS. *Disability and rehabilitation, 25*(20), 1168-1180.

Finucane, M. L. (2008). Emotion, affect, and risk communication with older adults: challenges and opportunities. *Journal of Risk Research, 11*(8), 983-997.

Fisher, B. J., & Specht, D. K. (1999). Successful aging and creativity in later life. *Journal of aging studies, 13*(4), 457-472.

Fletcher, J. (1960). The patient's right to die. *Harper's Magazine, 221*, 139-43.

Fooken, I. (1982). Patterns of health behavior, life satisfaction, and future time perspective in a group of old aged women: Data of "survivors" from a longitudinal study on aging. *International Journal of Behavioral Development, 5*(3), 367–390. https://doi.org/10.1177/016502548200500306

Fontaine, P.E. (1996). Exercise, fitness, and feeling well. *American Behavioral Science, 39*, 288–305.

Forbes, D. A., Finkelstein, S., Blake, C. M., Gibson, M., Morgan, D. G., Markle-Reid, M., …Thiessen, E. (2012). Knowledge exchange throughout the dementia care journey by Canadian rural community-based health care practitioners, persons with dementia, and their care partners: An interpretive descriptive study. *Rural and Remote Health, 12*(4), 2201-2201.

Fortinsky, R. H., & Downs, M. (2014). Optimizing person-centered transitions in the dementia journey: A comparison of national dementia strategies. *Health Affairs (Project Hope), 33*, 566 – 573. doi: 10.1377/hlthaff.2013.1304

Fowler, C., & Fisher, C.L. (2009). Attitudes toward decision making and aging, and preparation for future care needs. *Health Communication, 24*, 619–630. doi:10.1080/10410230903242226

Freedman, V. A., Kasper, J. D., & Spillman, B. C. (2017). Successful aging through successful accommodation with assistive devices. *Journals of Gerontology Series B: Psychological Sciences and Social Sciences, 72*(2), 300-309.

Friedman, C., & Rizzolo, M. C. (2016). Un/Paid labor: Medicaid home and community based services waivers that pay family as personal care providers. *Intellectual and Developmental Disabilities, 54*(4), 233-244. https://doi.org/10.1352/1934-9556-54.4.233

Fretz, B. R., Kluge, N. A., Ossana, S. M., Jones, S. M., & Merikangas, M. W. (1989). Intervention targets for reducing preretirement anxiety and depression. *Journal of Counseling Psychology, 36*(3), 301.

Freund, A. M., Nikitin, J., & Ritter, J. O. (2009). Psychological consequences of longevity: The increasing importance of self-regulation in old age. *Human Development, 52*(1), 1-37. doi:10.1159/000189213

Friedemann, M. L., Newman, F. L., Seff, L. R., & Dunlop, B. D. (2004). Planning for long-term care: Concept, definition, and measurement. *The Gerontologist, 44*(4), 520-530.

Funk, L. M. (2004). Who wants to be involved? Decision-making preferences among residents of long-term care facilities. *Canadian Journal on Aging/ La Revue canadienne du vieillissement, 23*(1), 47-58.

Gary, T. L., Safford, M. M., Gerzoff, R. B., Ettner, S. L., Karter, A. J., Beckles, G. L., & Brown, A. F. (2008). Perception of neighborhood problems, health behaviors, and diabetes outcomes among adults with diabetes in managed care: The Translating Research into Action for Diabetes (TRIAD) study. *Diabetes Care, 31*(2), 273-278.

Gaugler, J. E., & Kane, R. L. (Eds.). (2015). *Family caregiving in the new normal.* Academic Press.

Gaugler JE, Reese M, Tanler R. Care to Plan: An Online Tool That Offers Tailored Support to Dementia Caregivers. Gerontologist. 2016 Dec;56(6):1161-1174. doi: 10.1093/geront/gnv150. Epub 2015 Nov 23.

Gerst, K., & Burr, J.A. (2008). Planning for end-of-life care: Black-white differences in the completion of advance directives. *Research on Aging, 30,* 428–449.

Gessert, C. E., Forbes, S., & Bern-Klug, M. (2001). Planning end-of-life care for patients with dementia: Roles of families and health professionals. *OMEGA - Journal of Death and Dying, 42*(4), 273–291. https://doi.org/10.2190/2MT2-5GYU-GXVV-95NE

Gilleard, C., & Higgs, P. (2011). Ageing abjection and embodiment in the fourth age. *Journal of Aging Studies, 25*(2), 135-142.

Gilroy, R. (2008). Places that support human flourishing: Lessons from later life. *Planning Theory & Practice, 9*(2), 145-163.

Girling, L. M., & Morgan, L. A. (2014). Older women discuss planning for future care needs: An explanatory framework. *Journal of Aging and Health*, *26*(5), 724-749.

Glass Jr, J. C., & Kilpatrick, B. B. (1998). Financial planning for retirement: An imperative for baby boomer women. *Educational Gerontology: An International Quarterly*, *24*(6), 595-617.

Golden, A. G., Corvea, M. H., Dang, S., Llorente, M., & Silverman, M. A. (2009). Assessing advance directives in the homebound elderly. *American Journal of Hospice and Palliative Medicine*, *26*(1), 13-17.

Gonzales, E., & Nowell, W. B. (2017). Social capital and unretirement: Exploring the bonding, bridging, and linking aspects of social relationships. *Research on Aging*, *39*(10), 1100-1117.

Grable, J. E., & Lytton, R. H. (2003). The development of a risk assessment instrument: A follow-up study. *Financial services review*, *12*(3).

Greenglass, E. R., & Fiksenbaum, L. (2009). Proactive coping, positive affect, and well-being: Testing for mediation using path analysis. *European psychologist*, *14*(1), 29-39.

Greenglass, E.R., Fiksenbaum, L., & Eaton, J. (2006). The relationship between coping, social support, functional disability, and depression in the elderly. *Anxiety, Stress, and Coping: An International Journal*, *19*, 15–31.

Greenwald M. [Accessed August 2009]; These Four Walls… Americans 45+ talk about home and community. 2003 Available at http://research.aarp.org.

Groger, L., & Mayberry, P. S. (2001). Caring too much? Cultural lag in African Americans' perceptions of filial responsibilities. *Journal of Cross-Cultural Gerontology*, *16*(1), 21-39.

Guo, M., Kim, S., & Dong, X. (2019). Sense of filial obligation and caregiving burdens among Chinese immigrants in the United States. *Journal of the American Geriatrics Society*, *67*(S3), S564-S570.

Ha, J. H., & Pai, M. (2012). Do personality traits moderate the impact of care receipt on end-of-life care planning?. *The Gerontologist*, *52*(6), 759-769.

Hayes, C. L., & Parker, M. (1993). Overview of the literature on pre-retirement planning for women. *Journal of Women & Aging*, *4*(4), 1-18.

Hayes-Roth, B., & Hayes-Roth, F. (1979). A cognitive model of planning. *Cognitive science*, *3*(4), 275-310.

Heckhausen, J., & Schulz, R. (1995). A life-span theory of control. *Psychological Review*, *102*(2), 284.

Heckhausen, J., Wrosch, C., & Schulz, R. (2013). A lines-of-defense model for managing health threats: A review. *Gerontology, 59*(5), 438-447.

Hershey, D. A., Brown, C. E., Jacobs-Lawson, J. M., & Jackson, J. (2001). Retirees' perceptions of important retirement decisions. *The Southwestern Journal on Aging, 16,* 91-100.

Hershey, D.A., Jacobs-Lawson, J.M., McArdle, J.J., Hamagami, F. (2007) Psychological foundations of financial planning for retirement. *Journal of Adult Development, 14,* 26–36. doi:10.1007/s10804-007-9028-1

Hershey, D.A. & Mowen, J.C. (2000) Psychological determinants of financial preparedness for retirement. *Gerontologist, 40,* 687–697. doi:10.1093/geront/40.6.687

Heyman, D., & Jeffers, (1965). Observations on the extent of concern and planning by the aged, for possible chronic illness. *Journal of the American Geriatrics Society, 13(2),*152-159.

Hillcoat-Nallétamby, S., & Ogg, J. I. M. (2014). Moving beyond 'ageing in place': older people's dislikes about their home and neighbourhood environments as a motive for wishing to move. *Ageing & Society, 34*(10), 1771-1796.

Hirschman, K. B., Kapo, J. M., & Karlawish, J. H. (2008). Identifying the factors that facilitate or hinder advance planning by persons with dementia. *Alzheimer disease and associated disorders, 22*(3), 293.

Hong, M., & Kim, K. (2020). Advance care planning among ethnic/racial minority older adults: Prevalence of and factors associated with informal talks, durable power of attorney for health care, and living will. *Ethnicity & Health, 1.* doi:10.1080/13557858.2020.1734778

Hong, M., Yi, E. H., Johnson, K. J., & Adamek, M. E. (2018). Facilitators and barriers for advance care planning among ethnic and racial minorities in the US: A systematic review of the current literature. *Journal of Immigrant and Minority Health, 20*(5), 1277-1287.

Hutteman, R., Hennecke, M., Orth, U., Reitz, A. K., & Specht, J. (2014). Developmental tasks as a framework to study personality development in adulthood and old age. *European Journal of Personality, 28*(3), 267-278.

Jacobs-Lawson, J. M., & Hershey, D. A. (2005). Influence of future time perspective, financial knowledge, and financial risk tolerance on retirement saving behaviors. *Financial Services Review-Greenwich-, 14*(4), 331.

Jacobs-Lawson, J. M., Hershey, D. A., & Neukam, K. A. (2004). Gender differences in factors that influence time spent planning for retirement. *Journal of*

Women & Aging, 16(3-4), 55-69.

Johnson, R. W., Toohey, D., & Joshua, M. Wiener. (2007). Meeting the long-term care needs of the baby boomers: how changing families will affect paid helpers and institutions. *Retirement Project Discussion Pape*r. Washington, DC: The Urban Institute. https://www.urban.org/sites/default/files/publi cation/43026/311451-Meeting-the-Long-Term-Care-Needs-of-the-Baby-Boomers.PDF

Jolanki, O., & Vilkko, A. (2015). The meaning of a "sense of community" in a Finnish senior co-housing community. *Journal of Housing for the Elderly, 29*(1-2), 111-125.

Kahana, E., Kelley-Moore, J., & Kahana, B. (2012). Proactive aging: A longitudinal study of stress, resources, agency, and well-being in late life. *Aging & Mental Health, 16*(4), 438-451.

Kearns, A., & Parkes, A. (2003). Living in and leaving poor neighbourhood conditions in England. *Housing Studies, 18*(6), 827-851.

Kelly, A. J., Fausset, C. B., Rogers, W., & Fisk, A. D. (2014). Responding to home maintenance challenge scenarios: the role of selection, optimization, and compensation in aging-in-place. *Journal of Applied Gerontology, 33*(8), 1018-1042.

Kim, J.E. & Moen P. (2001a). Is retirement good or bad for subjective well-being? *Current Directions in Psychological Science, 10*, 83–86

Kim J. E., Moen P., (2001b). Moving into retirement: Preparation and transitions in late midlife. In M. E. Lachman (ed). *Handbook of midlife development (pp.* 498-527). Wiley.

Kim, J. E., & Moen, P. (2002). Retirement transitions, gender, and psychological well-being: A life-course, ecological model. *The Journals of Gerontology Series B: Psychological Sciences and Social Sciences, 57*(3), P212-P222.

Kilty, K. M., & Behling, J. H. (1986). Retirement financial planning among professional workers. *The Gerontologist, 26*(5), 525-530.

Kojola, E., & Moen, P. (2016). No more lock-step retirement: Boomers' shifting meanings of work and retirement. *Journal of Aging Studies, 36*, 59-70.

Kornadt A.E., & Rothermund, K. (2014). Preparation for old age in different life domains: dimensions and age differences. *International Journal of Behavioral Development, 38*, 228–238. doi:10.1177/0165025413512065

Kornadt A.E., & Rothermund, K. (2015). Views on aging: domain-specific approaches and implications for developmental regulation. *Annual Review of*

*Gerontology & Geriatrics, 35,*121–144. doi:10.1891/0198-8794.35.121

Kornadt, A.E., Voss, P, Rothermund, K. (2015). Hope for the best—Prepare for the worst? Future self-views and preparation for age-related changes. *Psychology of Aging, 30,* 967–976. doi:10.1037/pag0000048.

Kornadt, A.E., Voss, P. & Rothermund, K. (2018). Subjective remaining lifetime and concreteness of the future as differential predictors of preparation for age-related changes. *European Journal of Ageing, 15,* 67–76. https://doi.org/10.1007/s10433-017-0426-

Kotter-Grühn, D., Grühn, D., & Smith, J. (2010). Predicting one's own death: the relationship between subjective and objective nearness to death in very old age. *European Journal of Ageing, 7,* 293–300. doi:10.1007/s10433-010-0165-1

Kulys, R., & Tobin, S. S. (1980). Interpreting the lack of future concerns among the elderly. *The International Journal of Aging and Human Development, 11*(2), 111-126.

Kutner, L. (1979). Euthanasia: Due process for death with dignity; the living will. *Indiana Law Journal (Bloomington), 54*(2), 201-228.

Lang, F. R., Baltes, P. B., & Wagner, G. G. (2007). Desired lifetime and end-of-life desires across adulthood from 20 to 90: A dual-source information model. *Journals of Gerontology - Series B Psychological Sciences and Social Sciences, 62*(5), P268-P276. doi:10.1093/geronb/62.5.P268

Lang, F. R., & Rupprecht, F. S. (2019). Motivation for longevity across the life span: An emerging issue. *Innovation in Aging, 3*(2), igz014. doi:10.1093/geroni/igz014

Laslett, P. (1989). A fresh map of life: the emergence of the third age. Weidenfeld & Nicolson.

Lee, M., Ryoo, J. H., Campbell, C., Hollen, P. J., & Williams, I. C. (2020). The impact of performing medical/nursing tasks at home among caregivers of individuals with cognitive impairment. *Journal of Applied Gerontology, 39*(11), 1203-1212. https://doi.org/10.1177/0733464819879014

Lee, J. E., Kim, D. L., Peitz, L., Kahana, E., & Kahana, B. (2019). Future care planning intervention with rural older adults. *Innovation in Aging, 3*(Supplement_1), S425-S425. doi:10.1093/geroni/igz038.1587

Lendon, J. P., Caffrey, C., & Lau, D. T. (2020). Advance directives state requirements, center practices, and participant prevalence in adult day services centers: Findings from the 2016 National Study of Long-Term Care Providers. *The Journals of Gerontology: Series B, Vol. XX (x),* 1–6.

Lerner, R. M., & Busch-Rossnagel, N. A. (1981). Individuals as producers of their development: A life-span perspective. New York: Academic Press.

Levi, B. H., Dellasega, C., Whitehead, M., & Green, M. J. (2010). What influences individuals to engage in advance care planning?. *American Journal of Hospice and Palliative Medicine, 27*(5), 306-312.

Levitt, R. (2013). *Aging in place: Facilitating choice and independence.* Evidence matters. Washington, DC: Office of Policy Development and Research, Department of Housing and Urban Development

Li, M. H., & Yang, Y. (2009). Determinants of problem solving, social support seeking, and avoidance: A path analytic model. *International Journal of Stress Management, 16*(3), 155.

Little, B. R., Salmela-Aro, K., & Phillips, S. D. (Eds.). (2017). *Personal project pursuit: Goals, action, and human flourishing.* Psychology Press.

Löckenhoff, C. E. (2012). Understanding retirement: The promise of life-span developmental frameworks. *European Journal of Ageing, 9*(3), 227-231. doi:10.1007/s10433-012-02419

Löckenhoff, C. E., & Carstensen, L. L. (2007). Aging, emotion, and health-related decision strategies: Motivational manipulations can reduce age differences. *Psychology and Aging, 22*(1), 134–46. https://doi.org/10.1037/0882-797 4.22.1.134

Long Term Care Group, Inc. & LifePlans, Inc. for U.S. Department of Health and Human Services. (2006). *Final report for phase I: Own Your Future campaign.*

Loretto, W., & Vickerstaff, S. (2013). The domestic and gendered context for retirement. *Human Relations, 66*(1), 65–86. https://doi.org/10.1177/ 0018726712455832

Lowenstein, A., Katz, R., & Gur-Yaish, N. (2007). Reciprocity in parent–child exchange and life satisfaction among the elderly: a cross-national perspective. *Journal of Social Issues, 63*(4), 865-883.

Lusardi, A. (1999). Information, expectations, and savings for retirement. In H. Aaron (Ed.), *Behavioral Dimensions of Retirement Economics* (pp. 81-115). Brookings Institution and Russell Sage Foundation.

Lusardi, A., & Mitchell, O. S. (2008). Planning and financial literacy: How do women fare? *American Economic Review, 98*(2), 413-17.

Lynn, J., & Teno, J. M. (1993). After the Patient Self-Determination Act The Need for Empirical Research on Formal Advance Directives. *The Hastings Center*

Report, 23(1), 20-24.

Mackinac Center for Public Policy. (2019). "A Brief Explanation of the Overton Window". Mackinac Center for Public Policy. Retrieved 22 November 2019 from https://www.mackinac.org/OvertonWindow

Markus, H., & Nurius, P. (1986). Possible selves. *American Psychologist, 41*(9), 954-969. doi:10.1037//0003-066X.41.9.954

Marsiske, M., Lang, F.R., Baltes, P.B., Baltes, M.M. (1995). Selective optimization with compensation: life-span perspectives on successful human development. In: W.J. & A. Grob (Eds.). *Control of human behavior, mental processes, and consciousness: Essays in honor of the 60th birthday of August Flammer* (pp. 35–77). Lawrence Erlbaum Associates.

Mather, M., & Carstensen, L. L. (2005). Aging and motivated cognition: The positivity effect in attention and memory. *Trends in cognitive sciences, 9*(10), 496-502.

Meriam, L. (1918). *Principles Governing the Retirement of Public Employees* (Vol. 25). New York: D. Appleton and Company.

Mitchell, S. L., Shaffer, M. L., Cohen, S., Hanson, L. C., Habtemariam, D., & Volandes, A. E. (2018). An advance care planning video decision support tool for nursing home residents with advanced dementia: a cluster randomized clinical trial. *JAMA Internal Medicine, 178*(7), 961-969.

Miyawaki, C. E. (2017). Association of filial responsibility, ethnicity, and acculturation among Japanese American family caregivers of older adults. *Journal of Applied Gerontology, 36*(3), 296-319.

Moses, S. A. (2011). Medi-Cal long-term care: Safety net or hammock. *San Francisco, CA: Pacific Research Institute*. Retrieved from http://centerltc.com/pubs/Medi-Cal_LTC--Safety_Net_or_Hammock.pdf

Muller, J. S., Hiekel, N., & Liefbroer, A. C. (2020). The long-term costs of family trajectories: Women's later-life employment and earnings across Europe. *Demography*, 1-28.

Muratore, A. M., & Earl, J. K. (2015). Improving retirement outcomes: The role of resources, pre-retirement planning and transition characteristics. *Ageing and Society, 35*(10), 2100.

Mynors-Wallis, L. M., Gath, D. H., Lloyd-Thomas, A. R., & Tomlinson, D. B. M. J. (1995). Randomised controlled trial comparing problem solving treatment with amitriptyline and placebo for major depression in primary care. *BMJ, 310*(6977), 441-445.

National Center for Health Statistics (2020). NCHS Fact Sheet: April 2020. Retrieved from https://www.cdc.gov/nchs/data/factsheets/factsheet_NVSS.pdf

National Council on Aging and John Hancock Mutual Life Insurance Company. (1999, March). Long-term care survey. Arlington, VA: National Council on Aging.

Neukam, K. A., & Hershey, D. A. (2003). Financial inhibition, financial activation, and saving for retirement. *Financial Services Review, 12*(1), 19.

Niu, G., Zhou, Y., & Gan, H. (2020). Financial literacy and retirement preparation in China. *Pacific-Basin Finance Journal, 59*, 101262.

Noone, J., Alpass, F., & Stephens, C. (2010). Do men and women differ in their retirement planning? Testing a theoretical model of gendered pathways to retirement preparation. *Research on Aging 32*, 715–738. doi:10.1177/0164027510383531

Noone, J., O'Loughlin, K., Kendig, H. (2012). Socioeconomic, psychological and demographic determinants of Australian baby boomers' financial planning for retirement. *Australas Journal of Ageing, 31*, 94–197. doi:10.1111/j.1741-6612.2012.00600.x

Noone, J., O'Loughlin, K., & Kendig, H. (2013). Australian baby boomers retiring 'early': Understanding the benefits of retirement preparation for involuntary and voluntary retirees. *Journal of Aging Studies, 27*(3), 207-217.

Noone, J.H., Stephens, C., Alpass, F.M. (2009) Preretirement planning and well-being in later life. *Research on Aging, 31*, 295–317. doi:10.1177/0164027508330718

Noone, J. H., Stephens, C., & Alpass, F. (2010). The process of Retirement Planning Scale (PRePS): Development and validation. *Psychological Assessment, 22*(3), 520.

Nurmi, J. (1992). Age differences in adult life goals, concerns, and their temporal extension: A life course approach to future-oriented motivation. *International Journal of Behavioral Development, 15*(4), 487-508. doi:10.1177/016502549201500404

Organisation for Economic Co-operation and Development (OECD) (2016). Household savings forecast (indicator). doi:10.1787/6ab4e1bd-en (Accessed on 30 November 2020)

O'Rand, A. M., & Henretta, J. C. (1982). Delayed career entry, industrial pension structure, and early retirement in a cohort of unmarried women. *American Sociological Review*, 365-373.

Oswald, F., & Rowles, G. D. (2006). *Beyond the relocation trauma in old age: New trends in today's elders' residential decisions.* In H.-W. Wahl, C. Tesch-Römer, & A. Hoff (Eds.), New Dynamics in Old Age: Environmental and Societal Perspectives (pp. 127-152). Amityville, New York: Baywood Publ.

Oswald, F., & Wahl, H-W. (2005). *Dimension of the meaning of home.* In G. D. Rowles & H. Chaudhury (Eds.), Home and identity in later life: International perspectives (pp. 21–45). New York, NY: Springer.

Ouwehand, C., De Ridder, D. T., & Bensing, J. M. (2007). A review of successful aging models: Proposing proactive coping as an important additional strategy. *Clinical psychology review, 27*(8), 873-884.

Ouwehand, C., De Ridder, D. T., & Bensing, J. M. (2008a). The characteristics of a potential goal threat predict attention and information-seeking in middle-aged and older adults. *Motivation and Emotion, 32*(2), 90-99.

Ouwehand, C., de Ridder, D. T., & Bensing, J. M. (2008b). Individual differences in the use of proactive coping strategies by middle-aged and older adults. *Personality and Individual Differences, 45*(1), 28-33.

Owen, A. M. (1997). Cognitive planning in humans: neuropsychological, neuroanatomical and neuropharmacological perspectives. *Progress in neurobiology, 53*(4), 431-450.

Quine, S., Wells, Y., De Vaus, D., & Kendig, H. (2007). When choice in retirement decisions is missing: Qualitative and quantitative findings of impact on well-being. *Australasian Journal on Ageing, 26*(4), 173-179.

Parker, A. M., Bruine de Bruin, W., Yoong, J., & Willis, R. (2012). Inappropriate confidence and retirement planning: Four studies with a national sample. *Journal of Behavioral Decision Making, 25*, 382–389.

Penningroth, S. L., & Scott, W. D. (2012). Age-related differences in goals: Testing predictions from selection, optimization, and compensation theory and socioemotional selectivity theory. *The International Journal of Aging and Human Development, 74*(2), 87-111.

Perkins, K. (1995). Social [in] security: Retirement planning for women. *Journal of Women & Aging, 7*(1-2), 37-53.

Perry, T. E., & Thiels, J. F. (2016). Moving as a family affair: Applying the SOC model to older adults and their kinship networks. *Journal of Family Social Work, 19*(2), 74–99. https://doi.org/10.1080/10522158.2016.1157845

Petkoska, J., & Earl, J.K. (2009). Understanding the influence of demographic and psychological variables on retirement planning. *Psychological Aging, 24,*

245–251. doi:10.1037/a0014096

Pinquart, M., & Sörensen, S. (2002). Psychological outcomes of preparation for future care needs. *Journal of Applied Gerontology, 21,* 452–470. doi:10.11 77/073346402237632

Pinquart, M., & Sörensen, S. (2005). Ethnic Differences in Stressors, Resources, and Psychological Outcomes of Family Caregiving: A Meta-Analysis. *Gerontologist, 45*(1), 90-106.

Point-du-Jour, J. & Sörensen, S (2009). Improving problem-solving and future planning among older adults with macular degeneration. Paper presented at the Symposium on "Adaptation to Vision Loss: A Synthesis of Recent Empirical Work," 62nd Annual Scientific Meeting of the Gerontological Society of America, Atlanta, GA.

Prenda, K.M., & Lachman, M.E. (2001.) Planning for the future: a life management strategy for increasing control and life satisfaction in adulthood. *Psychological Aging, 16,* 206–216. doi:10.1037//0882-7974.16.2.206

Prendergast, T. J. (2001). Advance care planning: pitfalls, progress, promise. *Critical Care Medicine, 29*(2), N34-N39.

Preston, C., Drydakis, N., Forwood, S., Hughes, S., & Meads, C. (2019). What are the structural barriers to planning for later life? A scoping review of the literature. *Social Inclusion, 7*(3), 17-26.

Quick, H. E., & Moen, P. (1998). Gender, employment and retirement quality: A life course approach to the differential experiences of men and women. *Journal of occupational health psychology, 3*(1), 44.

Rabow, M. W., Hauser, J. M., & Adams, J. (2004). Supporting family caregivers at the end of life: They don't know what they don't know. *Journal of the American Medical Association* (JAMA) 291(4): 483-91.

Ramsaroop, S.D., Reid, M.C, & Adelman, R.D. *(2007).* Completing an advance directive in the primary care setting: What do we need for success? *Journal of the American Geriatric Society, 55, 277–283.*

Rao, J.K., Anderson, L.A., Lin, F., & Laux, J.P. (2014) Completion of advance directives among U.S. consumers. *American Journal of Preventative Medicine, 46* (1), 65-70.

Rebok, G. W. (1989). Plans, Action, & Transactions in Solving Everyday Problems. In J.D.Sinnott, (Ed.) *Everyday problem solving: Theory & application. New York: Praeger.*

Regan, T. (2017). Millennials Beat Baby Boomers in Long-Term Care Planning. *Senior Housing News,*

Reitzes, D. C., & Mutran, E. J. (2004). The transition to retirement: Stages and factors that influence retirement adjustment. *The International Journal of Aging and Human Development, 59*(1), 63-84.

Reuter, T., Ziegelmann, J. P., Wiedemann, A. U., Lippke, S., Schüz, B., & Aiken, L. S. (2010). Planning bridges the intention–behaviour gap: Age makes a difference and strategy use explains why. *Psychology and Health, 25*(7), 873-887.

Rhodes, R. L., Elwood, B., Lee, S. C., Tiro, J. A., Halm, E. A., & Skinner, C. S. (2017). The desires of their hearts: the multidisciplinary perspectives of African Americans on end-of-life care in the African American community. *American Journal of Hospice and Palliative Medicine, 34*(6), 510-517.

Richter, K. P., Langel, S., Fawcett, S. B., Paine-Andrews, A., Biehler, L., & Manning, R. (1995). Promoting the use of advance directives: an empirical study. *Archives of family medicine, 4*(7), 609.

Riediger, M., Freund, A. M., & Baltes, P. B. (2005). Managing life through personal goals: Intergoal facilitation and intensity of goal pursuit in younger and older adulthood. *The Journals of Gerontology Series B: Psychological Sciences and Social Sciences, 60*(2), P84-P91.

Robison, J. T., & Moen, P. (2000). A life-course perspective on housing expectations and shifts in late midlife. *Research on Aging, 22*(5), 499-532.

Robison, J., Shugrue, N., Fortinsky, R. H., & Gruman, C. (2014). Long-term supports and services planning for the future: Implications from a statewide survey of baby boomers and older adults. *The Gerontologist, 54*(2), 297-313.

Rosenkoetter, M. M., & Garris, J. M. (2001). Retirement planning, use of time, and psychosocial adjustment. *Issues in Mental Health Nursing, 22*(7), 703-722.

Roth, D. L., Haley, W. E., Wadley, V. G., Clay, O. J., & Howard, G. (2007). Race and gender differences in perceived caregiver availability for community-dwelling middle-aged and older adults. *The Gerontologist, 47*(6), 721-729.

Rowe, J. W., & Kahn, R. L. (1997). Successful aging. *The Gerontologist, 37*(4), 433-440. doi:10.1093/geront/37.4.433

Roy N, Dubé R, Després C, Freitas A, Legaré, F (2018) .Choosing between staying at home or moving: A systematic review of factors influencing housing decisions among frail older adults. *PLoS ONE, 13*(1): e0189266

Rurup, M. L., Onwuteaka-Philipsen, B. D., van der Heide, A., van der Wal, G., & Deeg, D. J. (2006). Frequency and determinants of advance directives concerning end-of-life care in The Netherlands. *Social science & medicine, 62*(6), 1552-1563.

Sabia, J. J. (2008). There's no place like home: A hazard model analysis of aging in place among older homeowners in the PSID. *Research on Aging, 30*(1), 3-35.

Sanders, C., & Schmitter-Edgecombe, M. (2012). Identifying the nature of impairment in planning ability with normal aging. *Journal of Clinical and Experimental Neuropsychology, 34*(7), 724-737.

Schans, D. (2008). 'They ought to do this for their parents': perceptions of filial obligations among immigrant and Dutch older people. *Ageing and Society, 28*(1), 49.

Schindler, I., & Staudinger, U. M. (2008). Obligatory and optional personal life investments in old and very old age: Validation and functional relations. *Motivation and Emotion, 32*(1), 23-36. doi:10.1007/s11031-007-9078-5

Schmid, T., Brandt, M., & Haberkern, K. (2011). Gendered support to older parents: do welfare states matter?. *European Journal of Ageing, 9*(1), 39–50. https://doi.org/10.1007/s10433-011-0197-1

Schnitzspahn, K. M., & Kliegel, M. (2009). Age effects in prospective memory performance within older adults: The paradoxical impact of implementation intentions. *European Journal of Ageing, 6*(2), 147-155.

Scholnick, E. K., & Friedman, S. L. (1993). Planning in context: Developmental and situational considerations. *International Journal of Behavioral Development, 16*(2), 145-167.

Schulz, R., Beach, S. R., Friedman, E. M., Martsolf, G. R., Rodakowski, J., & James III, A. E. (2018). Changing structures and processes to support family caregivers of seriously ill patients. *Journal of palliative medicine, 21*(S2), S-36. https://doi.org/10.1089/jpm.2017.0437

Schulz, R., & Czaja, S. J. (2018). Family caregiving: A vision for the future. *The American Journal of Geriatric Psychiatry, 26*(3), 358-363. https://doi.org/10.1016/j.jagp.2017.06.023

Slovic, P., Finucane, M. L., Peters, E., & MacGregor, D. G. (2004). Risk as analysis and risk as feelings: Some thoughts about affect, reason, risk, and rationality. *Risk Analysis: An International Journal, 24*(2), 311-322.

Social Security Administration. 2020. "A summary of the 2020 annual reports." http://www.ssa.gov/oact/trsum/.

Soichit, N., & Khophai, N. (2017). Local government organizations in Kalasin province with improving saving behaviors of the middle-aged people in preparation for aging society. *Chophayom Journal, 28*(3), 113-118.

Soldo, B.J., Mitchell, O.S., Tfaily, R. & McCabe, J.F. (2006). Cross-cohort differences in health on the verge of retirement. NBER Working Paper 12762. National Bureau of Economic Research, Inc. https://ideas.repec.org/p/nbr/nberwo/12762.html

Song, Y., Yan, E.C.W., & Sörensen. S. (2016). Family support and preparation for future care needs among urban Chinese baby boomers. *Journal of Gerontology: Social Sciences.* DOI: 10.1093/geronb/gbw062

Song, Y., Yan, E.C.W., & Sörensen. S. (2017). The effects of familism on intended care arrangements in the process of preparing for future care among one-child parents in urban China. *Ageing and Society, 37*(7), 1416-1434. DOI:10.1017/S0144686X16000349

Sörensen, S. (2019, November). Perspectives on Age-Related and Future Care Planning. *Discussion for* Future care planning and end-of-life care decision making: Individual and social influences. Presentation at the 71st Annual Meeting of the Gerontological Society of America, Austin, TX.

Sörensen, S., Duberstein, P. R., Chapman, B., Lyness, J. M., & Pinquart, M. (2008). How are personality traits related to preparation for future care needs in older adults? *The Journals of Gerontology. Series B, Psychological Sciences and Social Sciences, 63*(6), P328-P336. doi:10.1093/geronb/63.6.p328

Sörensen, S., Hirsch, J. K., & Lyness, L.M. (2014). Optimism and planning for future care needs among older adults. *Geropsych: The Journal of Gerontopsychology and Geriatric Psychiatry*, 27 (1), 5-22. DOI: 10.1024/1662-9647/a000099

Sörensen, S., Mak, W. & Pinquart, M. (2011). Planning and decision-making for care transitions. In Special Issue by P. Dilworth-Anderson, & M. Palmer (eds.), Pathways through the Transitions of Care for Older Adults. Annual Review of Gerontology and Geriatrics, *31*(1), 111-142(32)

Sörensen, S., Mak, W., Chapman, B.P., Duberstein, P.R., & Lyness, J.M. (2012). The relationship of preparation for future care and depression and anxiety in primary care patients: A two-year follow-up. *American Journal of Geriatric Psychiatry, 20*(10), 887–894. DOI: 10.1097/JGP.0b013e31822ccd8c. PMC3458161.

Sörensen, S. & Pinquart, M. (2000a). Preparation for future care needs by West and East German seniors. *Journal of Gerontology: Social Sciences, 55B* (6), S357-S367.

Sörensen, S. & Pinquart, M. (2000b). Preparation for future care needs: Styles of preparation used by older Eastern German, United States, and Canadian women. *Journal of Cross-Cultural Gerontology, 15* (4), 349-381.

Sörensen, S. & Pinquart. M. (2000c). Vulnerability and access to resources as predictors of preparation for future care needs in the elderly. *Journal of Aging and Health, 12* (3), 275-300.

Sörensen, S., & Zarit, S. H. (1996). Preparation for caregiving: A study of multi-generation families. *International Journal of Aging and Human Development, 42* (1), 43-63. doi: 10.1080/14616730210123102

Sörensen, S., Webster, J. D., & Roggman, L. A. (2002). Adult attachment and preparing to provide care for older relatives. *Attachment & Human Development, 4*(1), 84-106.

Sörensen, S., White, K., Mak, W., Zanibbi, K., Tang, W., O'Hearn, A., Hegel, M.T. (2015). The Macular Degeneration and Aging Study: Design and research protocol of a randomized trial for a psychosocial intervention with macular degeneration patients. *Contemporary Clinical Trials, 42*, 68-77. DOI: 10.1016/j.cct.2015.03.007

Sörensen, S., White, K., Sterns, G., Zanibbi, K. (2014, November). Effects of a preventive problem-solving intervention on macular degeneration patients' planning and depression. Presentation at the Symposium "Age-Related Vision Loss: Understanding and Addressing the Consequences". In *67th Annual Scientific Meeting of the Gerontological Society of America.* doi:10.2147/OPTH.S80489

Sörensen, S., & Zarit, S. H. (1996). Preparation for caregiving: A study of multi-generation families. *International Journal of Aging and Human Development, 42* (1), 43-63. doi: 10.1080/14616730210123102

Southerland, J., Slawson, D.L., Pack, R., Sörensen, S., Lyness, J.M., & Hirsch, J.K. (2016). Trait hope and preparation for future care needs among older adult primary care patients. *Clinical Gerontologist, 39* (2), 117-126. DOI: 10.1080/07317115.2015.1120254

Spitze, G., & Ward, R. (2000). Gender, marriage, and expectations for personal care. *Research on Aging, 22*(5), 451-469.

Stack, C. B., & Burton, L. M. (1993). Kinscripts. *Journal of Comparative Family Studies, 24*(2), 157-170.

Stawski, R. S., Hershey, D. A., & Jacobs-Lawson, J. M. (2007). Goal clarity and financial planning activities as determinants of retirement savings contributions. *The International Journal of Aging and Human Development, 64*(1), 13-32.

Steele, M., Pinquart, M., & Sorensen, S. (2003). Preparation dimensions and styles in long-term care. *Clinical Gerontologist, 26*(3-4), 105-122.

Sterns, H. L., Subich, L. M., Brown, S. D., & Lent, R. W. (2005). Counseling for retirement. *Career development and counseling: Putting theory and research to work,* 506-521.

Stones, D., & Gullifer, J. (2016). 'At home it's just so much easier to be yourself': Older adults' perceptions of ageing in place. *Ageing and Society, 36*(3), 449-481. doi:10.1017/S01446

Street, D., Desai, S. (2011). Planning for old age. In Settersten, R. A., Angel, J. L. (Eds.), *Handbook of Sociology of Aging* (pp. 379–397). New York, NY: Springer.

Strough, J., Berg, C. A., & Sansone, C. (1996). Goals for solving everyday problems across the life span: Age and gender differences in the salience of interpersonal concerns. *Developmental Psychology, 32*(6), 1106.

Sudore, R. L., & Fried, T. R. (2010). Redefining the "planning" in advance care planning: preparing for end-of-life decision making. *Annals of internal medicine, 153*(4), 256-261.

Szanton, S. L., Leff, B., Wolff, J. L., Roberts, L., & Gitlin, L. N. (2016). Home-based care program reduces disability and promotes aging in place. *Health Affairs (Project Hope), 35*(9), 1558–1563. doi:10.1377/hlthaff.2016.0140.

Tamborini, C. R., Iams, H. M., & Whitman, K. (2009). Marital history, race, and social security spouse and widow benefit eligibility in the United States. *Research on Aging, 31*(5), 577-605.

Tamborini, C. R., & Purcell, P. (2016). Women's household preparation for retirement at young and mid-adulthood: Differences by children and marital status. *Journal of Family and Economic Issues, 37*(2), 226-241.

Tell, E. J., & Cutler, J. A. (2011). A national long-term care awareness campaign: A case study in social marketing. *Cases in Public Health Communication & Marketing, 5,* 75-110.

Tulle-Winton, E. (1999). Growing old and resistance: towards a new cultural economy of old age?. *Ageing & Society, 19*(3), 281-299.

Topa, G., Moriano, J. A., Depolo, M., Alcover, C. M., & Morales, J. F. (2009). Antecedents and consequences of retirement planning and decision-making: A meta-analysis and model. *Journal of Vocational Behavior, 75*(1), 38-55.

Triplett, P., Black, B. S., Phillips, H., Richardson Fahrendorf, S., Schwartz, J., Angelino, A. F., ... & Rabins, P. V. (2008). Content of advance directives for individuals with advanced dementia. *Journal of Aging and Health, 20*(5), 583-596.

Turner, M. J., Bailey, W. C., & Scott, J. P. (1994). Factors influencing attitude toward retirement and retirement planning among midlife university employees. *Journal of Applied Gerontology, 13*(2), 143-156.

Unterrainer, J. M., & Owen, A. M. (2006). Planning and problem solving: from neuropsychology to functional neuroimaging. *Journal of Physiology-Paris, 99*(4-6), 308-317.

US Department of Health and Human Services (2017). Find your path forward: How much care will you need? Retrieved from https://longtermcare.acl.gov/the-basics/how-much-care-will-you-need.html .Accessed 8/12/2020.

Verbrugge, L. M., & Jette, A. M. (1994). The disablement process. *Social Science and Medicine, 38*(1) l-14.

Vincent, G. K., & Velkoff, V. A. (2010). The next four decades: The older population in the United States: 2010 to 2050 (No. 1138). US Department of Commerce, Economics and Statistics Administration, US Census Bureau.

Vora, P. P., & McGinnis, J. D. (2000). The asset allocation decision in retirement: Lessons from dollar-cost averaging. *Financial Services Review, 9*(1), 47-63.

Wakefield, M. A., Loken, B., & Hornik, R. C. (2010). Use of mass media campaigns to change health behaviour. *The Lancet, 376*(9748), 1261-1271.

Walz, H. S., & Mitchell, T. E. (2007). Adult Children and Their Parents' Expectations of Future Elder Care Needs. *Journal of Aging and Health, 19*(3), 482–499. https://doi.org/10.1177/0898264307300184

Wang, M., & Shi, J. (2014). Psychological research on retirement. *Annual review of psychology, 65*, 209-233.

Wangmo, T. (2010). Changing expectations of care among older Tibetans living in India and Switzerland. *Ageing and society, 30*(5), 879.

Watson, J., & McNaughton, M. (2007). Gender differences in risk aversion and expected retirement benefits. *Financial Analysts Journal, 63*(4), 52-62.

Weathers, E., O'Caoimh, R., Cornally, N., Fitzgerald, C., Kearns, T., Coffey, A., ... & Molloy, D. W. (2016). Advance care planning: a systematic review of randomised controlled trials conducted with older adults. *Maturitas, 91*, 101-109.

Wetherell, J. L., Reynolds, C. A., Gatz, M., & Pedersen, N. L. (2002). Anxiety, cognitive performance, and cognitive decline in normal aging. *The Journals of Gerontology Series B: Psychological Sciences and Social Sciences, 57*(3), P246-P255.

Whitlatch, C. J., Judge, K., Zarit, S. H., & Femia, E. (2006). Dyadic intervention for family caregivers and care receivers in early-stage dementia. *The Gerontologist, 46*(5), 688-694. https://doi.org/10.1093/geront/46.5.688

Williams, R.A., Brody, B.L., Thomas, R.G., Kaplan, R.M., & Brown, S.I. (1998). The psychosocial impact of macular degeneration. *Archives of Ophthalmology, 116*(4), 514-520.

Wolff, J. L., Feder, J., & Schulz, R. (2016). Supporting family caregivers of older Americans. *New England Journal of Medicine, 375*(26), 2513-2515.

Wolff, J. L., Spillman, B. C., Freedman, V. A., & Kasper, J. D. (2016). A national profile of family and unpaid caregivers who assist older adults with health care activities. *JAMA Internal Medicine, 176*(3), 372-379.

Wolff, J. L., Spillman, B. C., Freedman, V. A., Kasper, J. D. (2016). A national profile of family and unpaid caregivers who assist older adults with health care activities. *JAMA Internal Medicine, 176*(3), 372-379. doi:10.1001/jamaintern med.2015.7664

Wolinsky, F.D., Stump, T.E., & Clarke, D.O. (1995). Antecedents and consequences of physical activity and exercise among older adults. *Gerontologist, 35*, 451–62.

World Health Organization. (2015). *World report on ageing and health*. World Health Organization.

Yadav, K. N., Gabler, N., Cooney, E., Kent, S., Kim, J., Herbst, N., ... & Courtright, K. R. (2017). Prevalence Of Advance Directives In The United States: A Systematic Review. *Presentation in Updates In Advanced Care Planning And End Of Life Care In Respiratory And Critical Illness* (pp. A4633-A4633) at the American Thoracic Society, 2017.

Dickemper, J., & Yakoboski, P. (1997). *Increased saving but little planning: Results of the 1997 Retirement Confidence Survey (Issue Brief No. 191). Washington*. DC: Employee Benefit Research Institute. https://www.ebri.org/publica tions/research-publications/issue-briefs/content/increased-saving-but-lit tle-planning-results-of-the-1997-retirement-confidence-survey-102

Yeung, D.Y. (2013). Is pre-retirement planning always good? An exploratory study of retirement adjustment among Hong Kong Chinese retirees. *Aging and Mental Health, 17*, 386–393. doi:10.1080/13607863.2012.732036

Yeung, D. Y., & Zhou, X. (2017). Planning for retirement: Longitudinal effect on retirement resources and post-retirement well-being. *Frontiers in psychology, 8*(1300), 1-14.

Zanjari, N., Sharifian Sani, M., Hosseini Chavoshi, M., Rafiey, H., & Mohammadi Shahboulaghi, F. (2016). Perceptions of successful ageing among Iranian elders: insights from a qualitative study. *The International Journal of Aging and Human Development, 83*(4), 381-401.

Zaremba, J. F. (1987). Death with dignity: Implementing one's right to die. *University of Detroit Law Review, 64*(3), 557-577.

Notes

1. 43% built up saving; 45% learned about pension and Social Security benefits and thought about whether to move or age in place; 58% bought their own home; 56% developed hobbies and other leisure time activities; 33% prepared a will; 56% made sure they had medical care available.

2. Tulle-Winton's provocative interpretation of this phenomenon suggests that there is a link between recent "gerontological pronouncements about what it is possible to achieve in old age" and the regulation of populations and the "disciplining of individual bodies" into age-segregated spaces. The author sees the lack of planning for housing transitions as a form of resistance to societal processes that shun old bodies, emphasizing their loss of cultural value. "However, it is recast within a framework of obligations for social actors to avoid social and cultural segregation, thus seeming to act both as goal and as evaluation of later life and of old people's ability to adapt to changing biographical and environmental conditions" (p.296).

3. We thank the anonymous reviewers for this additional consideration.

Featured Titles from Westphalia Press

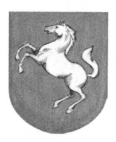

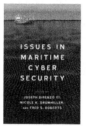

Issues in Maritime Cyber Security Edited by Nicole K. Drumhiller, Fred S. Roberts, Joseph DiRenzo III and Fred S. Roberts

While there is literature about the maritime transportation system, and about cyber security, to date there is very little literature on this converging area. This pioneering book is beneficial to a variety of audiences looking at risk analysis, national security, cyber threats, or maritime policy.

The Death Penalty in the Caribbean: Perspectives from the Police Edited by Wendell C. Wallace PhD

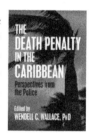

Two controversial topics, policing and the death penalty, are skillfully interwoven into one book in order to respond to this lacuna in the region. The book carries you through a disparate range of emotions, thoughts, frustrations, successes and views as espoused by police leaders throughout the Caribbean

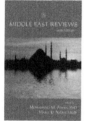

Middle East Reviews: Second Edition Edited by Mohammed M. Aman PhD and Mary Jo Aman MLIS

The book brings together reviews of books published on the Middle East and North Africa. It is a valuable addition to Middle East literature, and will provide an informative read for experts and non-experts on the MENA countries.

Unworkable Conservatism: Small Government, Freemarkets, and Impracticality by Max J. Skidmore

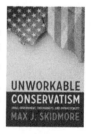

Unworkable Conservatism looks at what passes these days for "conservative" principles—small government, low taxes, minimal regulation—and demonstrates that they are not feasible under modern conditions.

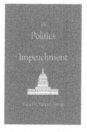

The Politics of Impeachment Edited by Margaret Tseng

This edited volume addresses the increased political nature of impeachment. It is meant to be a wide overview of impeachment on the federal and state level, including: the politics of bringing impeachment articles forward, the politicized impeachment proceedings, the political nature of how one conducts oneself during the proceedings and the political fallout afterwards.

Demand the Impossible: Essays in History as Activism
Edited by Nathan Wuertenberg and William Horne

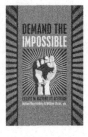

Demand the Impossible asks scholars what they can do to help solve present-day crises. The twelve essays in this volume draw inspiration from present-day activists. They examine the role of history in shaping ongoing debates over monuments, racism, clean energy, health care, poverty, and the Democratic Party.

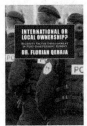

International or Local Ownership?: Security Sector Development in Post-Independent Kosovo
by Dr. Florian Qehaja

International or Local Ownership? contributes to the debate on the concept of local ownership in post-conflict settings, and discussions on international relations, peacebuilding, security and development studies.

Donald J. Trump's Presidency: International Perspectives
Edited by John Dixon and Max J. Skidmore

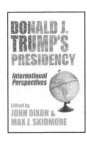

President Donald J. Trump's foreign policy rhetoric and actions become more understandable by reference to his personality traits, his worldview, and his view of the world. As such, his foreign policy emphasis was on American isolationism and economic nationalism.

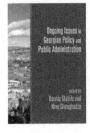

Ongoing Issues in Georgian Policy and Public Administration
Edited by Bonnie Stabile and Nino Ghonghadze

Thriving democracy and representative government depend upon a well functioning civil service, rich civic life and economic success. Georgia has been considered a top performer among countries in South Eastern Europe seeking to establish themselves in the post-Soviet era.

Poverty in America: Urban and Rural Inequality and Deprivation in the 21st Century
Edited by Max J. Skidmore

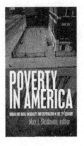

Poverty in America too often goes unnoticed, and disregarded. This perhaps results from America's general level of prosperity along with a fairly widespread notion that conditions inevitably are better in the USA than elsewhere. Political rhetoric frequently enforces such an erroneous notion.

westphaliapress.org

Made in the USA
Columbia, SC
23 April 2021